T0134405

Cardiac Magnetic Resonance Atlas

Yasmin Rustamova • Massimo Lombardi

Cardiac Magnetic Resonance Atlas

101 Clinical Cases

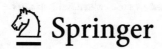 Springer

Yasmin Rustamova
Educational-Surgery Clinic
Azerbaijan Medical University
Baku
Azerbaijan

Massimo Lombardi
Multimodality Cardiac Imaging section
I.R.C.C.S. Policlinico San Donato
San Donato Milanese
Milan
Italy

ISBN 978-3-030-41832-8   ISBN 978-3-030-41830-4   (eBook)
https://doi.org/10.1007/978-3-030-41830-4

This Springer imprint is published by the registered company Springer Nature Switzerland AG
The registered company address is: Gewerbestrasse 11, 6330 Cham, Switzerland

Preface

This cardiac magnetic atlas was born to fill a gap between the existing textbooks in the field and the practical neediness of the single operator who is facing the individual diagnostic procedure. The atlas, in fact, aims to give the operator the diagnostic targets and the expected results in the most common cardiac pathologies affecting the patients undergoing a cardiac magnetic resonance examination. The atlas is comprehensive of 101 clinical cases covering the whole spectrum of adult cardiac pathologies. Because of space limitations the number of congenital heart disease and the vascular cases has been limited to the most common pathologies.

Each clinical case is accompanied by a descriptive card where the essential anamnestic details are provided. Similarly, the individual card is comprehensive of the main diagnostic findings in the specific case which is evaluated according to a quite monotonous acquisition flowchart. In each clinical case, the diagnostic procedure adheres to the suggestions of the main scientific societies (EACVI and SCMR) integrated with the personal experience of the operators, who are all trained according to the international certification processes.

All cases have been acquired using a high-performance 1.5 Tesla scanner equipped with a multichannel surface coil. The scanner is fully dedicated to cardiac activity and ruled by a strict quality control.

All cases are provided with a variable number of figures where the most relevant pathologic findings are illustrated. Cine images are synthetized by end-diastolic and end-systolic frames.

The online version is also provided with the relative movies.

In each card, the main scientific references are also provided. When it resulted impossible to represent the diagnostic background by a few relevant papers, the recent published textbook on cardiac MR which is part of the textbooks family of the EACVI has been suggested as generic reference.

The authors hope that this atlas will represent a true help for the operators who are daily challenged by difficult cases evaluated by this specific imaging modality which is gradually changing the diagnostic paradigm in cardiology.

Baku, Azerbaijan   Yasmin Rustamova
Milan, Italy   Massimo Lombardi

Technical Details

All patients were evaluated using a commercial 1.5T magnet, bore diameter of 70 cm, maximum gradient strength of 57 mT/m, and maximum slew rate of 264 (mT/m/ms).

All images were acquired in breath hold, after having optimized the sequence so that the patients were asked to stop breathing for no more than 10–12 s. When the acquisition was obtained during deep or superficial anesthesia, sequences were optimized accordingly, such as increasing the number of excitation. When the patient was assisted by an automatic respirator, images were acquired stopping the ventilation process.

In the presence of extrasystolic activity affecting the image quality, a pharmacological attempt has been done to regularize the cardiac rhythm adopting one of the following procedures:

(a) e.v. administration of atropine (up to 2 mg) when there was evidence that the extrasystolic activity was reduced by increasing the heart rate (e.g., during an ECG effort test)
(b) e.v. administration of xylocaine (up to 100 mg)
(c) Administration of flecainide (50 mg b.i.d.) in the 7–10 days preceding the examination

When necessary a Gd-based cyclic contrast agent has been administered i.v. at the dosage of 1.0–2.0 mmol/kg.

All pharmacological stresses were performed after β-blockers, calcium antagonists, nitrates, caffeine, theine, etc. washout (since 48–72 h before the test).

Anesthesiological approach:

1. Sedation: during continuous infusion of propofol (2–3 mg/kg/h)
2. General anesthesia: sevoflurane administered as a volatile anesthetic agent in a mixture of air and oxygen (0.5–5%)

Each acquisition sequence was optimized in each patient. Here, the typical values are reported:

Cine images: Steady-state free processing (SSFP): TR 55 ms, TE 1.60 ms, FA 60°. Number of segments optimized according to RR. Reconstruction phases 30 frames/beat. Reconstruction matrix 256 × 192 pixels and FOV 350 mm. Slice thickness 8 mm (in small children 6 mm), no gap.

Black blood images, proton density weighted: TR 1800 ms. TE 40 ms. Echo train 7 or according to the heart rate. FA 180°, FOV 400 mm, matrix 320 × 208 pixels.

Black blood images, T1w: TR <900 ms, TE 25 ms, echo train 8, FA 180°, FOV 320, matrix 320 × 208 pixels.

Black blood images, T2w: TR 2000 ms, TE 75 ms, echo train 6, FA 180°, FOV 300, matrix 256 × 208 pixels.

Three-dimensional contrast-enhanced angiography (CEMRA): TR 2.5 ms, TE 0.9 ms, FA 25°, FOV 400 mm, slices × slab 128, slice thickness 1.3 mm, contrast dose 1.5–2.0 mmol/kg, injected by a power injector at 2–2.5 ml/s.

Time-resolved 3D angiography: TR 2.5 ms, TE 0.9 ms, FA 28°, FOV 340 mm, slice thickness 1.3 mm, slices × slab 112, measurements 11, temporal resolution 3.5–4 s. Contrast dose 1.5–2.0 mmol/kg, injected by a power injector at 2–2.5 ml/s.

Late enhancement 2D, single slice: TR 1600 ms, TE 3.3 ms, FA 25°, FOV 400 mm, matrix 256 × 192 pixels, slice thickness 8 mm, TI optimized during acquisition.

Rapid single-breath-hold 3D late gadolinium enhancement cardiac MR: TR 700 ms or less according to heart rate, TE 1.1 ms, FA 25°, TI optimized, matrix 208 × 166, 10–12 slices, slice thickness 8 mm.

3D navigator fat at T2 prep: TR 309 ms, TE 1.53 ms, FA 90°, FOV 380 mm, matrix 256 × 256 pixels, slice thickness 0.8 mm, T2 prep duration 40 ms.

Phase contrast (flow images): TR 37 ms, TE 2.5 ms, slice thickness 6 mm, FOV 400 mm, matrix 192 × 170 pixels, FA 20°, acceleration factor 2, VENC optimized.

Perfusion images (GRE-IR): TR 175 ms, TE 1.29 ms, slice thickness 8 mm, FOV, matrix 160 × 112. Contrast agent 0.5–0.75 mmol/kg administered by a power injection in 3 s or less.

Mapping

Molli: TR 280 ms, TE 1.1 ms, slice thickness 8 mm, FA 35°, FOV 360 mm, matrix 256 × 256 pixels.

Sh Molli: TR 37 ms, TE 1 ms, FA 35°, slice thickness 8 mm, FOV 360 mm, matrix 192 × 192 pixels.

T2 mapping (true FISP): TR 193 ms, TE 1.03 ms, FA 70°, FOV 360 mm, matrix 192 × 144 pixels, slice thickness 8 mm.

T2∗ mapping GRE (heart): TR 700 ms, TE varying between 2.08 and 16.22 ms, FA 20°, matrix 256 × 154 pixels, thickness 10 mm.

T2∗ mapping GRE (liver): TR 200, TE varying between 0.93 and 14.24 ms, FA 23°, matrix 126 × 126 pixels, thickness 10 mm.

Acknowledgments

The authors would like to acknowledge the colleagues from the CMR lab of I.R.C.C:S. Policlinico San Donato, Milan, for their helpful collaboration and technical support. It is worthy of merit that without the work of Antonia Camporeale, Silvia Pica, and Francesca Pluchinotta the selection of cases, their analysis, and the synthesis of their clinical meaning would have been impossible.

Contents

Abbreviations

2D	Two dimensional
3D	Three dimensional
3D CEMRA	Three-dimensional contrast-enhanced magnetic resonance angiography
AMI	Acute myocardial infarction
CAD	Coronary artery disease
CMR	Cardiac magnetic resonance
DES	Drug eluting stent
ECV	Extracellular volume
EF	Ejection fraction
ER	Emergency rooms
FA	Flip angle
Gd	Gadolinium
LAD	Left anterior descending artery
LGE	Late gadolinium enhancement
LV	Left ventricle
LVED	Left ventricle end diastole
LVEF	Left ventricle ejection fraction
LVEDV	Left ventricle end diastolic volume
LVES	Left ventricle end systole
LVESV	Left ventricle end systolic volume
Molli	Modified look-locker inversion recovery
NYHA	New york heart association
PDw	Proton density weighted
PTCA	Primary transcutaneous coronary angioplasty
Qp/Qs	Ratio between pulmonary flow and systemic flow
RV	Right ventricle
RVED	Right ventricle end diastole
RVEDV	Right ventricle end diastolic volume
RVEF	Right ventricle ejection fraction
RVES	Right ventricle end systole
RVESV	Right ventricle end systolic volume
Sh-Molli	Shortened modified look-locker inversion recovery
SSFP:	Steady-state free precession
STEMI	ST elevation myocardial infarction
T1w	T1 weighted
T2w	T2 weighted
TAPSE	Tricuspid Annular Plane Excursion
TE	Time of echo
TOF	Tetralogy of Fallot
TR	Time of repetition
True FISP	(Fast imaging with steady-state precession)

List of Videos

1.1 Hypertrophic Cardiomyopathy

1.1.1 Hypertrophic Cardiomyopathy

Medical History Male, 46 y.o. Previous evidence of non-sustained ventricular tachycardia. Echocardiogram showing asymmetric myocardial hypertrophy.

CMR Flowchart Stack of cine images in short-axis view to evaluate biventricular volumes, segmental thickness of myocardium, and ventricular mass. T1 mapping (Sh_MOLLI pre- and postcontrast to measure ECV). Postcontrast LGE images.

Main CMR Findings Normal biventricular regional and global function. Increased thickness at the level of the anterior proximal septum (28 mm). All the other segments have normal thickness. Normal ventricular mass (Movie 1.1, Movie 1.2 and Movie 1.3). At LGE images intramyocardial fibrosis at the level of the thickened myocardium (<10% of the myocardial mass). Prolapse of anterior mitral leaflet while the posterior leaflet being hypoplastic. Increased ECV at the level of the hypertrophic segment (31%).

Conclusion Hypertrophic cardiomyopathy with evidence of intramyocardial fibrosis. Mitral valve dysplasia.

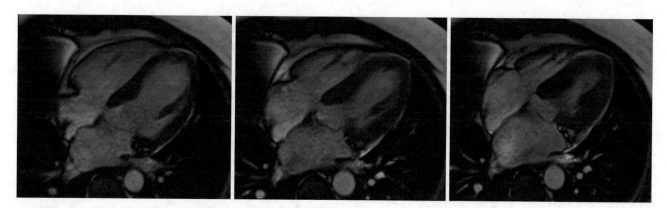

Fig. 1.1 SSFP cine images in horizontal long axis. During the diastolic phase (left panel) evidence of hypertrophy at the level of the interventricular septum. During the systolic phase (middle and right panels) evidence of abnormal movement of the anterior leaflet of mitral valve

Electronic Supplementary Material The online version of this chapter (https://doi.org/10.1007/978-3-030-41830-4_1) contains supplementary material, which is available to authorized users.

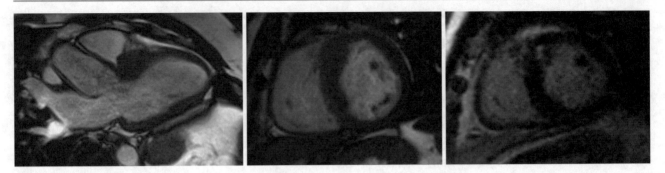

Fig. 1.2 In the left and middle panels SSFP cine images showing more clearly the segmental hypertrophy of myocardium. In the postcontrast LGE image (right panel) clear evidence of intramyocardial fibrosis which is disclosed by the uptake of the contrast agent

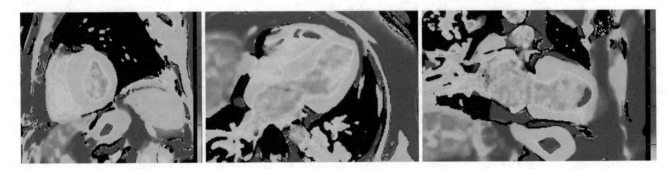

Fig. 1.3 T1 map images obtained in short axis (left panel), horizontal long axis (middle panel), and vertical long axis of the left ventricle (right panel)

1.1.2 Hypertrophic Cardiomyopathy with Signal Intensity Abnormalities

Medical History Male, 67 y.o. Already known as affected by obstructive hypertrophic cardiomyopathy and coronary artery disease and submitted to multiple percutaneous coronary angioplasty, the last 1 year earlier for stenting on posterior interventricular coronary artery. Currently reporting angina on effort and seldom at rest.

Patient submitted to CMR both for morpho-structural evaluation and detection of inducible ischemia by pharmacological stress.

CMR Flowchart Stack of SSFP cine images in short-axis view to evaluate biventricular function, segmental wall thickness, and myocardial mass. T2w images in short-axis view and horizontal and vertical long axis to detect the presence of myocardial edema. Perfusion images (three parallel short axes) baseline and during maximum vasodilatation (adenosine 140 µg/kg/min∗6 min). LGE images.

Main CMR Findings Normal biventricular function. Increased thickness of myocardium (max thickness at the level of midventricular anterior segment (20 mm)) (Movie 1.4, Movie 1.5 and Movie 1.6). In T2w images presence of increased signal at the level of anterior and anteroseptal segments and apical segments. During vasodilatation evidence of segmental hypoperfusion involving anterior midventricular segment and apical segments (Movie 1.7). In LGE images evidence of diffuse intramyocardial uptake at the level of anterior midventricular wall and apical segments.

Conclusion Hypertrophic cardiomyopathy with involvement of mid- and distal segments. Signal abnormalities of T2-weighted images are probably due to myocardial edema. Diffuse intramyocardial fibrosis mainly evident in the most thickened segments.

Large area of anterior and apical myocardial hypoperfusion during adenosine infusion. The lesions of coronary angiography do not justify the presence of such a large area of hypoperfusion, probably to be interpreted as a consequence of diffuse microvascular disease.

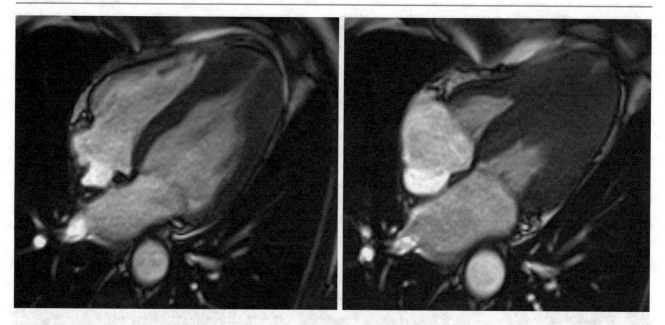

Fig. 1.4 SSFP cine images. Horizontal long axis. Left panel: end-diastolic frame. Right panel: end-systolic frame. Evidence of asymmetric hypertrophy involving the apical segments

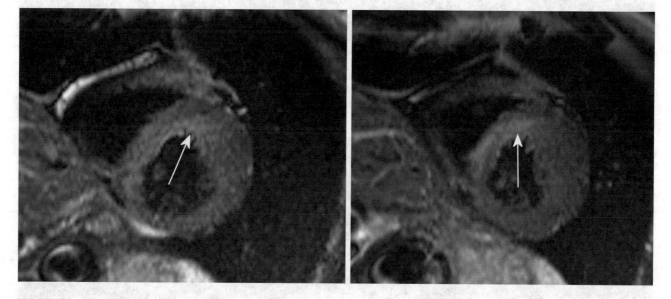

Fig. 1.5 T2-weighted images. Short-axis planes. Left panel: midventricular section. Right panel: apical projection. Arrows show the hyperintense areas due to the presence of intramyocardial edema

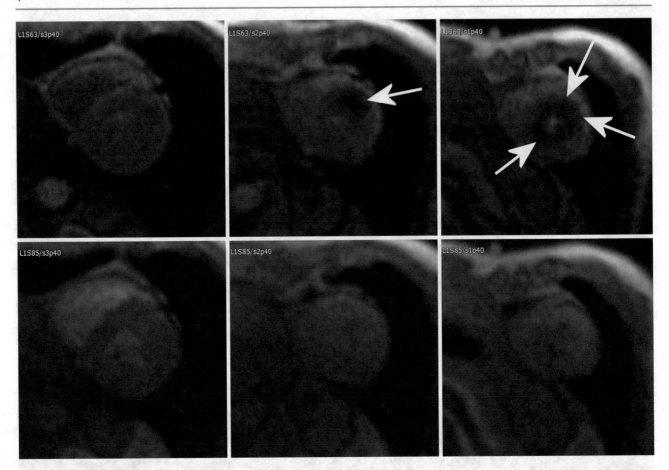

Fig. 1.6 Perfusion images. First-pass technique. Upper panels: three parallel slices in proximal, mid-, and apical positions (left to right). Upper panels: images obtained at maximum pharmacological vasodila-tation during adenosine infusion (140 µg/kg/min∗6 min). Lower panels: same planes in baseline conditions. Arrows show anterior midventricu-lar hypoperfusion and apical diffuse hypoperfusion during stress

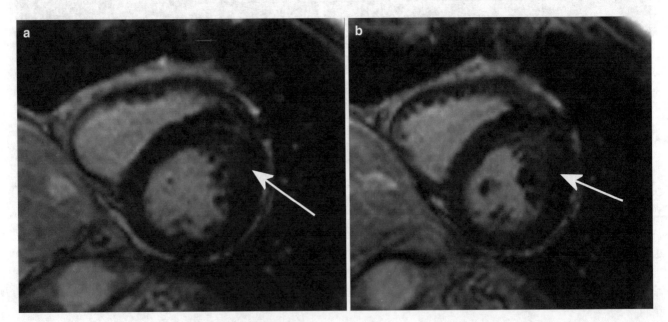

Fig. 1.7 LGE images obtained 10 minutes after the injection of c.a. six parallel slices in short-axis view (**a** and **b**: basal sections, **c** and **d**: mid-ventricular sections, **e** and **f**: apical sections). Arrows show the diffuse uptake of c.a. involving the anterior midventricular wall and the apical segments

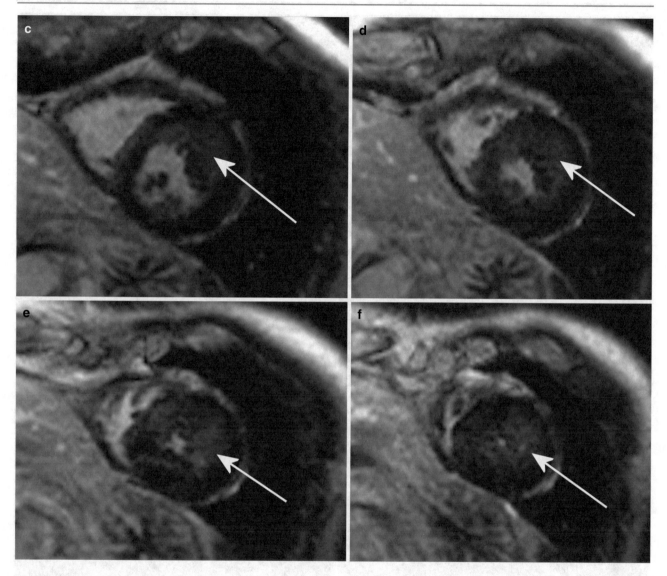

Fig. 1.7 (continued)

1.1.3 Obstructive Hypertrophic Cardiomyopathy

Medical History Male, 32 y.o. Palpitation and dizziness. At Echocardiography diagnosis of obstructive hypertrophic cardiomyopathy.

CMR Flowchart Stack of cine images in short-axis view to evaluate biventricular volumes, function, and myocardial thickness. Cine images in vertical and horizontal long-axis and three-chamber view. Postcontrast LGE images to evaluate the presence of intramyocardial fibrosis. T1 mapping images before and 15 min after the administration of 0.1 mmol/kg Gadolinium based c.a.

Main CMR Findings Normal biventricular regional and global function. Increased myocardial mass. Segmental hypertrophy involving the anterior and septal proximal segments. Maximum thickness 29 mm at the level of the anterior proximal segment (Movie 1.8, Movie 1.9 and Movie 1.10). Turbulence of flow at the level of the outflow tract. At LGE images patchy uptake of c.a. evident at the level of the anterior segment. Increased level of T1 mapping mainly at the anterior proximal segment with extracellular volume (ECV) expansion.

Hematocrit = 48%

Myocardial native T1 value: 1018 ms, postcontrast myocardial T1 value: 476 ms, native blood T1 value: 1518 ms, postcontrast blood T1 value: 390 ms, ECV: 30%.

Conclusion Hypertrophic cardiomyopathy with patchy fibrosis limited to the hypertrophic segments. Abnormal native T1 value with moderate enlargement of ECV.

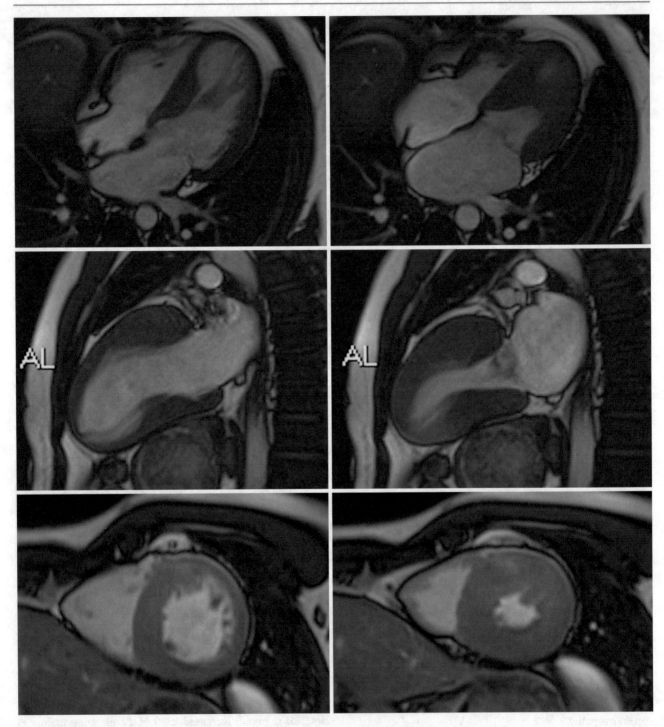

Fig. 1.8 SSFP cine images in horizontal long-axis plane (upper panels), vertical long-axis plane (middle panels), short-axis plane (lower panels), end-diastolic phase (left panels), and end-systolic phase (right panels). Evidence of hypertrophy at the level of proximal septal and anterior segments

Fig. 1.9   STIR T2w image in short-axis plane. The arrow shows an area of signal enhancement at the level of the anteroseptal proximal segment. This finding can be interpreted as an inflammatory process correlated to the hypertrophy (postischemic?)

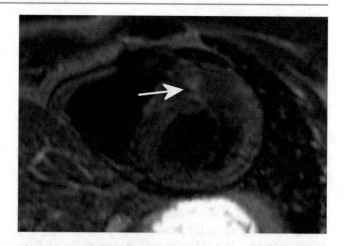

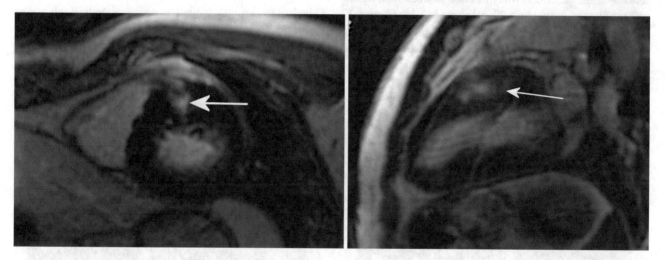

Fig. 1.10   Postcontrast LGE images in short-axis plane (left panel) and vertical long-axis plane (right panel). The arrows show the uptake of the contrast agent indicating a patchy intramyocardial fibrosis

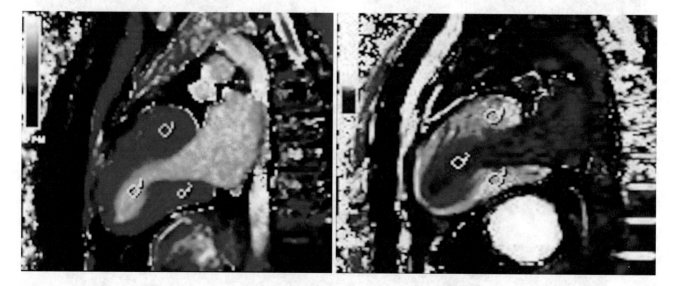

Fig. 1.11   T1 maps in vertical long-axis view. Left panel: native map. Right panel: postcontrast map (see text for explanation)

1.2   Dilated Cardiomyopathy

1.2.1   Primitive Dilated Cardiomyopathy

Medical History Male, 47 y.o. Overweight patient with family history of CAD. Two weeks before the examination admitted to the ER for epigastric pain and progressive dyspnea. Echocardiography showed dilated left ventricle with reduced systolic function (LVEF = 30%) and moderate mitral regurgitation. Invasive coronary angiography showed normal coronary arteries.

CMR Flowchart Stack of cine images in left ventricle short axis to cover the whole heart volume, for global and regional functional assessment; T2-weighted images to exclude inflammatory disease, precontrast T1 mapping to assess native T1 values; LGE images to confirm/exclude the presence of intramyocardial fibrosis and confirm/exclude inflammatory disease; postcontrast T1 mapping for ECV calculation.

Main CMR Findings Left ventricle volumes are at the upper limits of normal values. Global hypokinesia and severely reduced systolic function (LVEF = 20%) were found (Movie 1.11).

Volumes and function of the right ventricle within the normal range of values.

Images acquired after the administration of contrast media showed predominantly midwall enhancement at the level of the proximal interventricular septum and inferolateral wall.

Precontrast native T1 value: 941 (normal values 962 ± 25 ms) (Piechnik et al. JCMR 2013).

ECV: 32% (normal values: 25 ± 3%) (Fontana et al. JCMR 2012).

Conclusion Primitive dilated cardiomyopathy with severe reduction in systolic function. The presence of intramyocardial fibrosis has to be considered as a negative prognostic marker.

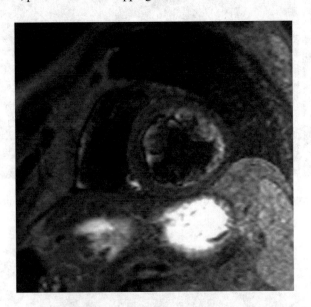

Fig. 1.12 Black blood T2-weighted image. Short-axis view of the left ventricle. No evidence of signal abnormalities

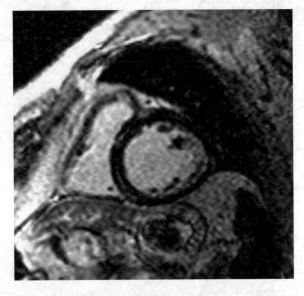

Fig. 1.13 LGE image. Intramyocardial linear uptake of the contrast agent. More evident at the level of the interventricular septum

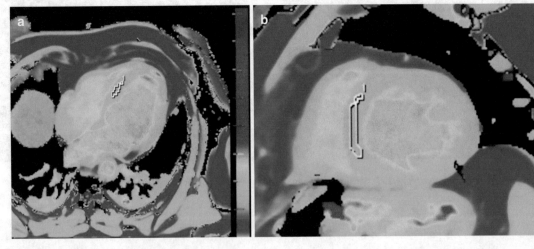

Fig. 1.14 (**a** and **b**) T1 mapping images in horizontal long axis and short axis of left ventricle. T1 values are collected at the level of the interventricular septum

1.2.2 Alcoholic Cardiomyopathy

Medical History Male, 37 y.o. Long-lasting alcohol abuse. Worsening dyspnea. Severe impairment of cardiac function at echocardiography. Suspect of infective disorder.

CMR Flowchart Stack of cine images in short-axis view to evaluate biventricular volumes and function. Stack of T2w images in short axis and vertical and horizontal long axis to assess the presence of myocardial edema. T1 mapping images before and after contrast agent administration (0.1 mmol/kg). LGE images to detect myocardial fibrosis.

Main CMR Findings Severe biventricular dilatation and impairment of global function (LV EF 21%, RV EF 24%) (Movie 1.12 and Movie 1.13). No signal abnormalities in T2w images. Increased value of native T1 (1080 ms) and increased extracellular volume (29%).

Conclusion Alcoholic cardiomyopathy with severe impairment of biventricular global function.

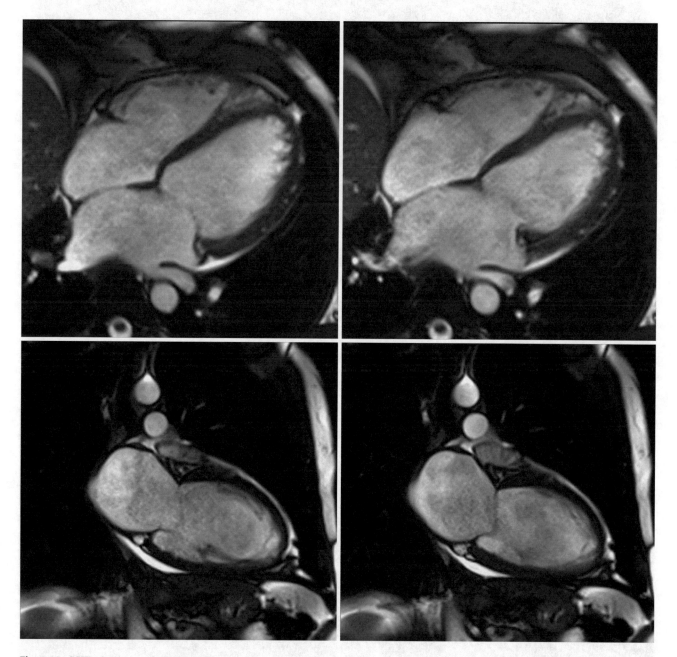

Fig. 1.15 SSFP cine images in horizontal long-axis (upper panels) and vertical long-axis plane (lower panels). Left panels in end diastole and right panels in end systole. Evidence of biventricular increase of volumes and severe impairment of global function

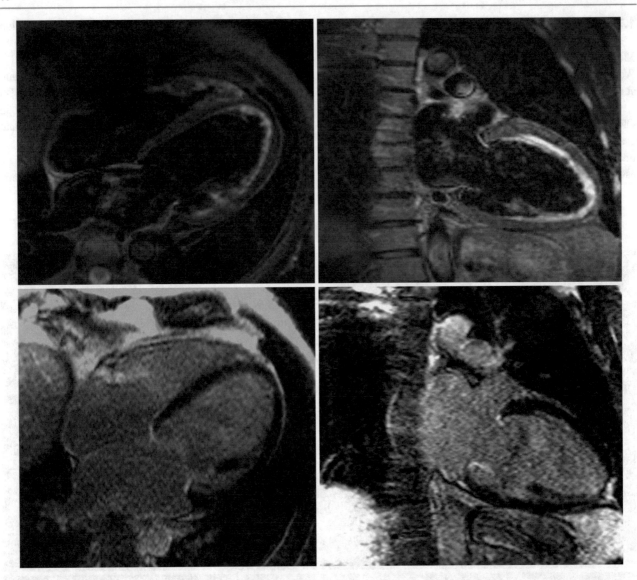

Fig. 1.16 Upper panels: T2w images. Lower panels: LGE images. Left panels: horizontal long axis. Right panels: vertical long axis. No evidence of signal abnormalities in T2w images. No contrast uptake in LGE images

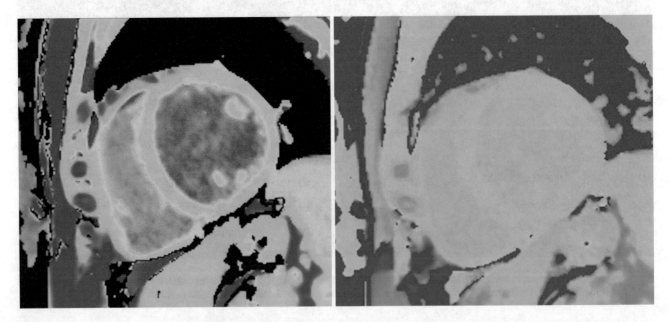

Fig. 1.17 T1 mapping images in midventricular short-axis view. Left panel: native T1 map. Right panel: postcontrast T1 map (0.1 mmol/kg)

1.3   Ventricular Noncompaction

1.3.1   Left Ventricular Noncompaction

Medical History Female, 19 y.o. Previous transcutaneous closure of interatrial defect. At Echocardiography slight reduction of global left ventricular function with globular morphology of apical segment.

CMR Flowchart Stack of cine in short-axis view to evaluate biventricular volumes and function. Cine images in oblique plan to evaluate the morphology of interatrial septum and to exclude/confirm the presence of residual shunt. Phase-contrast images at the level of the ascending aorta and at the level of pulmonary artery to evaluate the Qp/Qs. LGE images to characterize the myocardium.

Main CMR Findings Normal biventricular global function (EF 56%). Hypertrabeculation of the distal segments and mainly at the level of the apical septum. Noncompacted/compacted myocardium ratio: 4.0 (n.v. < 2.3), percentage of noncompacted with respect to the compacted myocardium: 24% (n.v. < 20%). Thinning of the apical segment of the interventricular septum (Movie 1.14 and Movie 1.15). In LGE images, transmural fibrosis of apical segment of the thinned interventricular septum. Presence of artifacts due to the metallic body of the interatrial closure device. No evidence of shunt: Qp/Qs = 1.

Conclusion Noncompacted myocardium. Previous interatrial defect. No residual shunt.

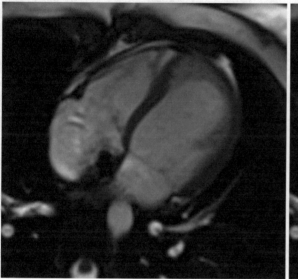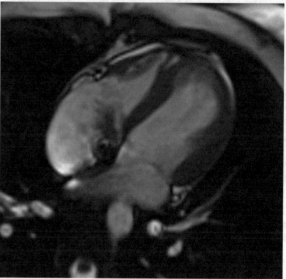

Fig. 1.18 SSFP cine images. Left panel: end diastolic frame. Right panel: end-systolic frame. Evidence of hypertrabeculation at the level of the apical part of the interventricular septum. With a noncompacted/compacted myocardium ratio of 4 (n.v. < 2.3) and a percentage of 24% with respect to the whole myocardial mass. Evidence of artifact at the level of the interatrial septum where an umbrella was previously positioned for closure of the atrial septal defect

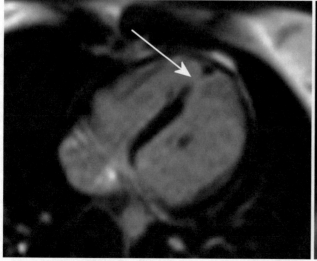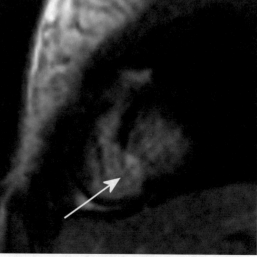

Fig. 1.19 LGE images obtained 10 min after the injection of gadolinium-based contrast agent (0.2 mmol/kg). Evidence of uptake at the level of the apical part of the interventricular septum (arrows). Left panel: horizontal long-axis view. Right panel: short-axis view

1.3.2 Biventricular Noncompaction

Medical History Female, 19 y.o. Previous diagnosis of aneurysm of the interatrial septum without evidence of shunt. At Echocardiography slight reduction of global left ventricular function with globular morphology of apical segment.

CMR Flowchart Stack of cine in short-axis view to evaluate biventricular volumes and function. Cine images in oblique plan to evaluate the morphology of the heart and to measure the ratio between the noncompacted and the compacted tissue. LGE images to characterize the myocardium.

Main CMR Findings Slight reduction of LV global function (EF 50%). Hypertrabeculation of both the left and the right ventricle. Noncompacted/compacted myocardium ratio: 3.5 (n.v. < 2.3), percentage of noncompacted with respect to the compacted myocardium: 34% (n.v. < 20%). Diffuse thinning of the compacted tissue (Movie 1.16 and Movie 1.17). In LGE images, no evidence of myocardial fibrosis.

Conclusion Biventricular noncompacted myocardium.

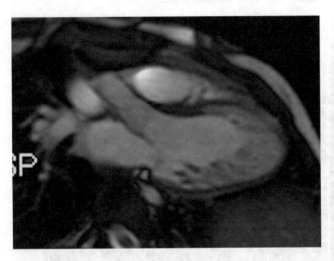

Fig. 1.20 SSFP cine images. Vertical long axis. End-diastolic frame showing an abnormal representation of intraventricular trabeculation with a pathologic ratio between noncompacted and compacted myocardium

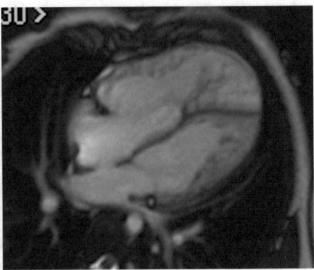

Fig. 1.21 SSFP cine images. Horizontal long axis. End-diastolic frame showing an abnormal representation of intraventricular trabeculation both inside the left and the right ventricles

1.4 Ventricular Dysplasia

1.4.1 Arrhythmogenic Right-Ventricle Dysplasia

Medical History Male, 9 y.o. Right-ventricle dilatation at transthoracic Echocardiography.

CMR Flowchart Stack of cine images in short-axis view to evaluate biventricular volumes and function. Stack of cine mages in para-axial plane to evaluate the right-ventricle regional kinesis. LGE images both in short axis of the heart and in par-axial plane for a better view of the right-ventricle free wall.

Main CMR Findings Left-ventricle volume within limits and normal global function (EF 65%). Presence of a multiple dyskinetic area at the level of the right-ventricle free wall (Movie 1.18 and Movie 1.19). In LGE images area of fibrosis in correspondence of the right-ventricle dyskinetic area.

Conclusion Right-ventricle dysplasia.

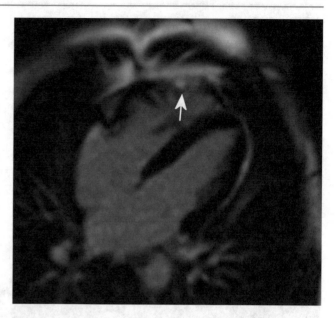

Fig. 1.23 LGE image in paraxial plane. Evidence of an area of contrast uptake (arrow) suggesting an area of fibrous substitution

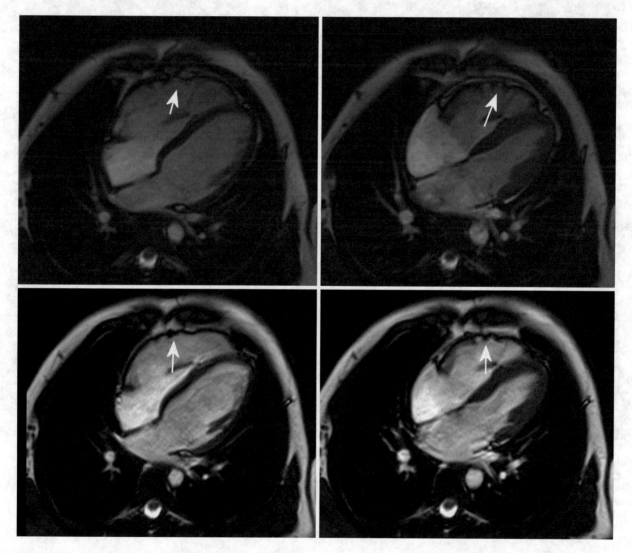

Fig. 1.22 SSFP cine images in two contiguous horizontal planes to evaluate the regional function of the right-ventricle free wall. Evidence of multiple pseudo-aneurisms which are more evident during the sys-tolic phase (right panels) but still clearly detectable during the diastolic phase (left panels)

1.4.2 Arrhythmogenic Biventricular Dysplasia

Medical History Male, 17 y.o. Minor ECG abnormalities (V1–V4 negative T wave), ventricular extra beats. Asymptomatic. Diagnostic suspect of Arrhythmogenic Right Ventricle Dysplasia (ARVD).

CMR Flowchart Stack of cine images in short-axis view to evaluate biventricular volumes and function. Cine images in para-axial plane to evaluate the right-ventricle free wall. Proton density weighted images both in short-axis view and para-axial plane. Same planes are utilized to obtain LGE images 10 min after the injection of a bolus of contrast agent (0.2 mmol/kg).

Main CMR Findings Right-ventricle enlargement (132 ml/m^2) with a global EF of 45%. Multiple segmental wall motion abnormalities both at the level of the left and of the right ventricles (Movie 1.20, Movie 1.21 and Movie 1.22). Multiple areas of fat infiltration mainly at the level of the left-ventricle lateral segments. Multiple areas of uptake of the contrast agent at LGE images.

Conclusion Biventricular dysplasia (probably arrhythmogenic).

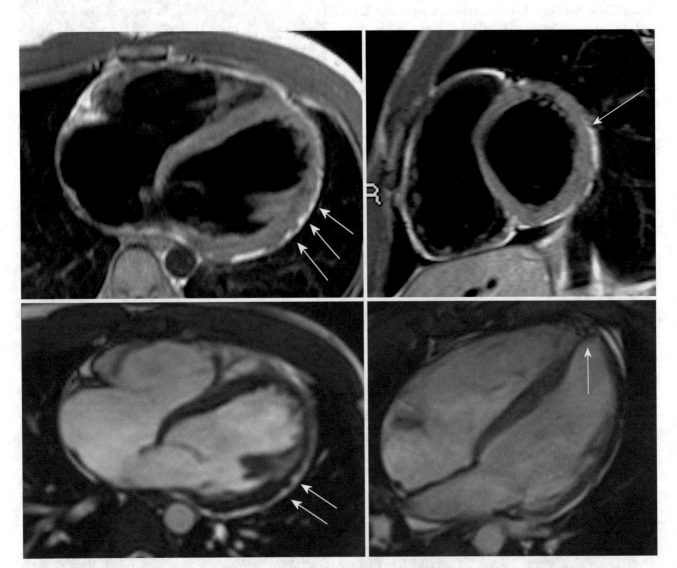

Fig. 1.24 PDw images in axial plane (upper left panel) and short axis (right upper panel). The arrows show the multiple areas of fat infiltration mainly at the level of the lateral wall of left ventricle. Still frame of a cine sequence in axial plane (lower left panel) showing multiple morphologic irregularity at the level of the lateral wall of the left ventricle presumably due to the fat infiltration (arrows). The still frame from a cine sequence obtained in horizontal long axis shows thinning of the interventricular septum in its apical segment with aneurismatic movement (arrow) (see Movie 1.20)

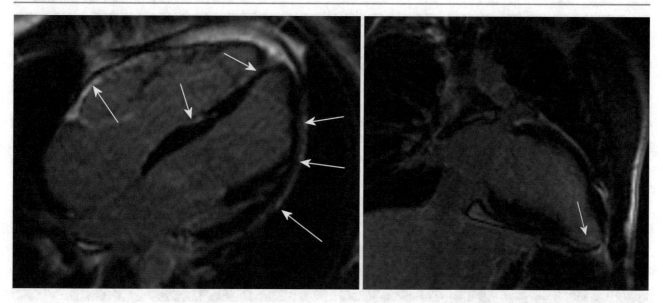

Fig. 1.25 LGE images in horizontal long axis (left panel) and vertical long axis (right panel). The arrows show multiple areas of fibrous infiltration

1.4.3 Arrhythmogenic Left-Ventricle Dominant Dysplasia

Medical History Female, 17 y.o. History of palpitation.

CMR Flowchart Stack of cine images in short-axis view to evaluate biventricular volumes and function. Black blood images PDw in short axis and long axis. Black blood images PDw with fat saturation in short axis and long axis. LGE images after the administration of a bolus of contrast agent (0.2 mmol/kg).

Main CMR Findings Normal biventricular regional and global function. Normal thickness of left ventricle walls (Movie 1.23). In black blood images and LGE images presence of multiple areas of myocardial substitution by fat and fibrofatty tissue.

Conclusion Left-ventricle dominant dysplasia.

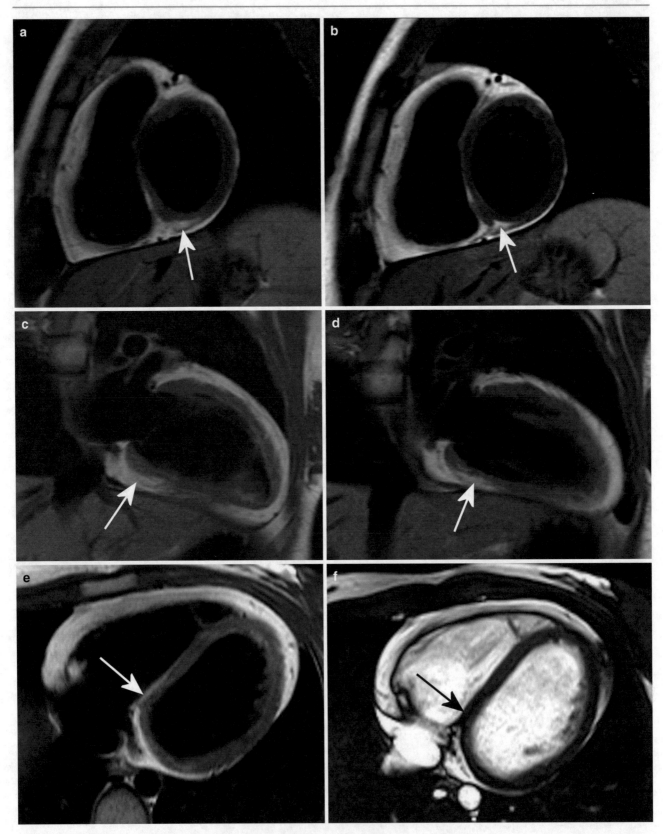

Fig. 1.26 Panels **a** and **b**: Black blood proton density weighted images. Short-axis view of the heart. Evidence of fatty infiltration at the level of inferior wall (arrows). Panels **c** and **d**: Black blood proton density weighted images. Vertical long axis of the left ventricle. Evidence of fatty infiltration at the level of inferior wall (arrows). Panel **e**: Black blood proton density weighted image in axial plane. Panel f: SSFP cine images in axial plane. End-diastolic frames. Evidence of fatty infiltration at the level of proximal septal wall (arrows)

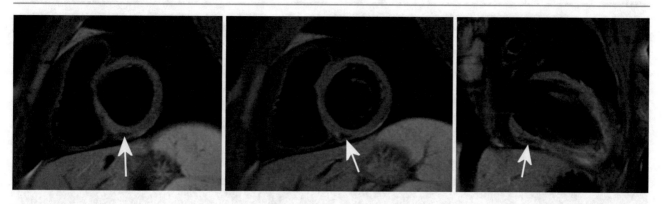

Fig. 1.27 Black blood proton density weighted images with fat suppression. Left and middle panels: short-axis view of the heart. Right panel: vertical long-axis view. Arrows show the area of fatty infiltration at the level of inferior wall.

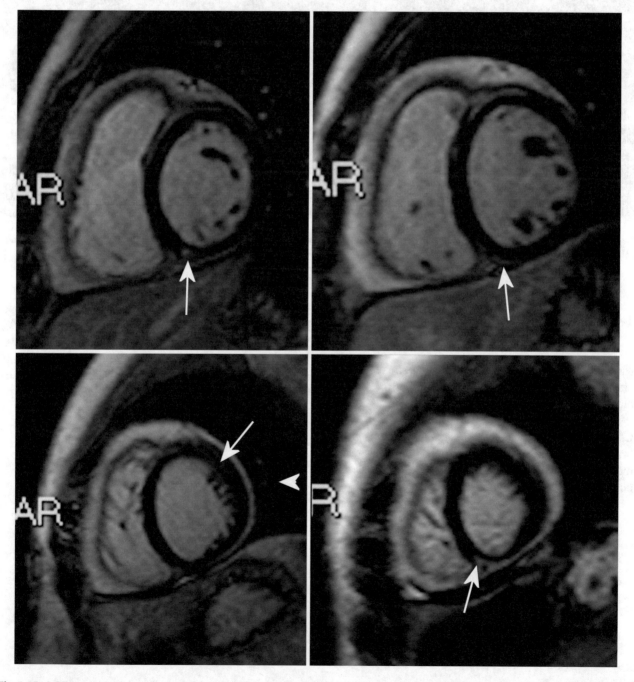

Fig. 1.28 LGE images in short-axis view of the heart. Four parallel planes. Arrows show the most evident areas of c.a. uptake

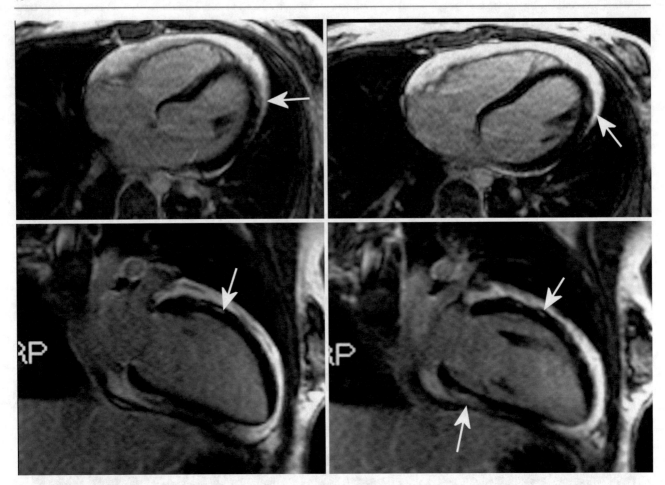

Fig. 1.29 LGE images in two horizontal long axes (upper panels) and two vertical long axes (lower panels) of the heart. Arrows show the most evident areas of c.a. uptake

1.4.4 Morphologically Dysplastic Left-Ventricle

Medical History Female, 38 y.o. Previous stroke. Previous closure of interatrial defect. Recent episode of transient diplopia.

CMR Flowchart Stack of cine images in short-axis view to evaluate biventricular volumes and function. Stack of cine mages in para-axial plane to evaluate the left-ventricle morphology. LGE images.

Main CMR Findings Left-ventricle volume at upper limit with slight reduction of global function (EF 48%). Presence of a large dyskinetic area with the morphology of large diverticulum in communication with the main left-ventricle cavity (Movie 1.24, Movie 1.25 and Movie 1.26). Normal right ventricle. In LGE images large area of fibrosis in correspondence of the dysplastic area.

Conclusion Morphologically Dysplastic Left-Ventricle.

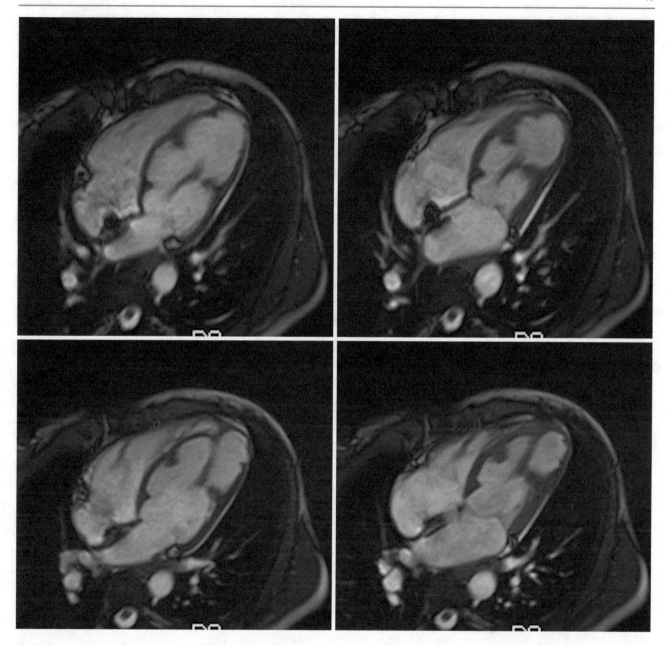

Fig. 1.30 SSFP cine images in two parallel horizontal long axis views of the heart. Evidence of a large dysplastic diverticulum at the apical level of the left ventricle whose inner cavity is in large communication with the main left-ventricle cavity. Evidence of metallic artifact at the level of the interatrial septum due to the presence of the umbrella device (left panels: diastolic phase; right panels: systolic phase)

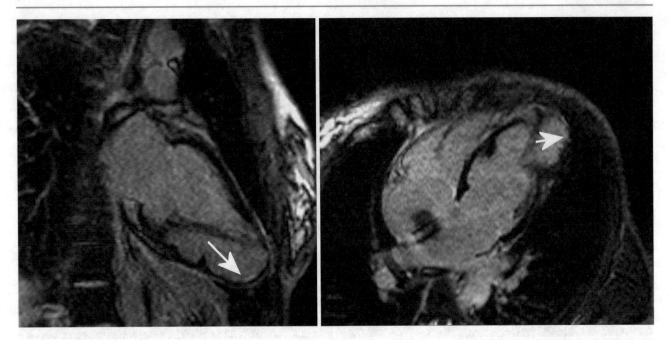

Fig. 1.31 LGE images in vertical long axis (left panel) and in horizontal long axis (right panel). Evidence of myocardial fibrosis at the level of the diverticulum (arrows). Evidence of metallic artifact at the level of the interatrial septum due to the presence of the umbrella device

1.5 Cardiac Involvement in Neurologic Disorders

1.5.1 Cardiac Involvement in Friedreich Ataxia

Medical History Male, 38 y.o. Patient affected by Friedreich ataxia. No history of cardiac involvement.

CMR Flowchart Stack of cine images in short-axis view to evaluate wall thickness and biventricular volumes and func-

tion. Stack of images in black blood proton density weighted in short axis view. Stack of LGE images in short axis view.

Main CMR Findings Left-ventricle volume within the normal limits. Moderate reduction of left-ventricle global function. Segmental hypertrophy mainly involving the interventricular septum (max thickness 16 mm) (Movie 1.27). In LGE images area of fibrosis at the level of the inferolateral segments.

Conclusion Cardiac involvement in a patient with Friedreich ataxia.

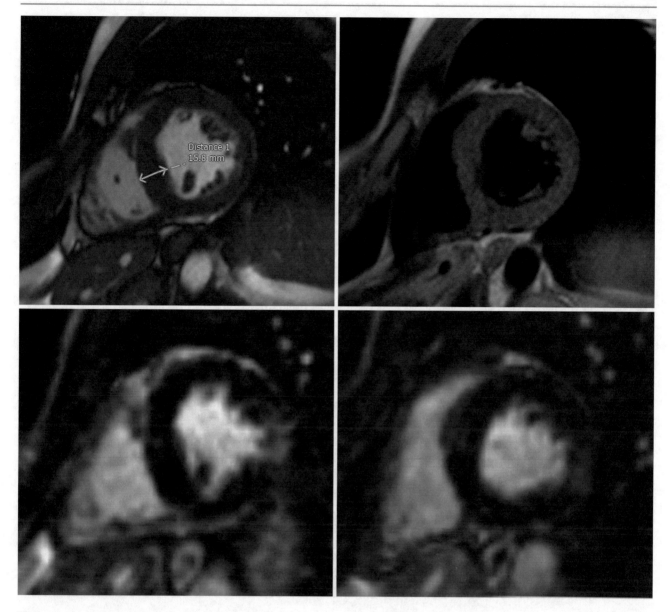

Fig. 1.32 Upper left panel: diastolic frame from a cine SSFP sequence in short axis of the heart. Evidence of segmental hypertrophy involving mainly the inferoseptal segment. Upper right panel: black blood PDw image in short-axis view of the same patient. No abnormality detected. Lower panels: LGE images with evidence of uptake of the contrast agent at the level of the inferolateral segment

1.5.2   Cardiac Involvement in Steinert Dystrophy

Medical History Male, 17 y.o. Affected by Steinert myodystrophy. Suspected involvement of the heart.

CMR Flowchart Stack of cine images in short-axis view to evaluate biventricular volumes, function, and wall thickness. Stack of T2w images. T1 mapping before and 15 min after c.a. administration (0.1 mmol/kg). LGE images.

Main CMR Findings Left-ventricle volumes and global function normal, right-ventricle volumes and function normal (Movie 1.28). No pathologic findings in T2w images. Normal myocardial native T1 values. Presence of pericardial and epicardial contrast uptake.

Conclusion Findings compatible with the diagnosis of Steinert myodystrophy.

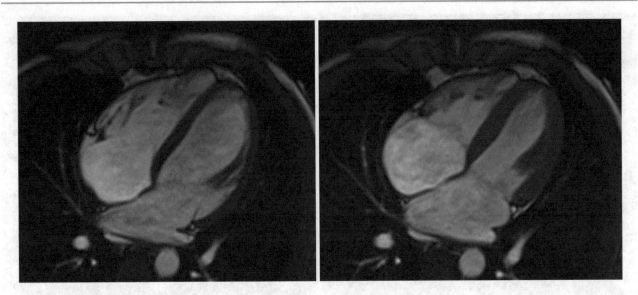

Fig. 1.33 SSFP cine images. Left panel: diastolic frame. Right panel: systolic frame. Evidence of normal regional and global function

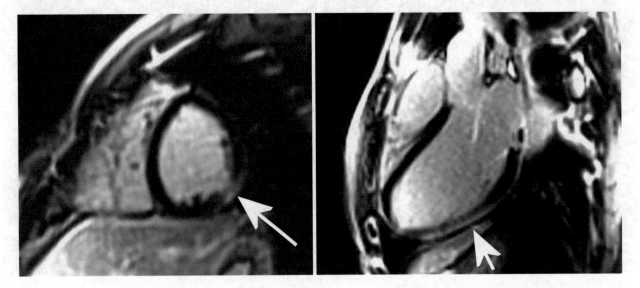

Fig. 1.34 LGE images. Left panel: short-axis view of the heart. Right panel: vertical long axis. The arrow shows the pericardial and subepicardial contrast uptake

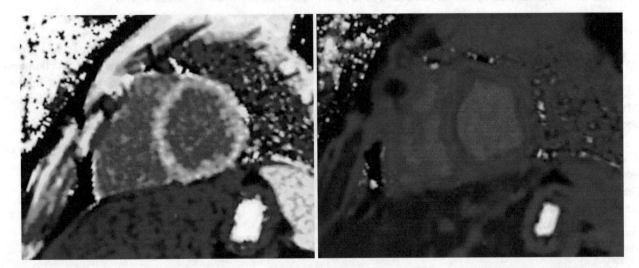

Fig. 1.35 T1 mapping Molli images in midventricular short-axis view. Left panel: native T1 map (1021 ± 55 ms). Right panel: postcontrast T1 map (634 ± 23 ms)

1.6   Infiltrative and Storage Cardiomyopathies

1.6.1   Cardiac Involvement in Anderson-Fabry Disease

Medical History Male, 53 y.o. Previous stroke. Genetic positive for Anderson-Fabry disease. Under enzymatic therapy. Hypertrophy at Echocardiography.

CMR Flowchart Stack of cine images in short-axis view to evaluate biventricular volumes, function, and wall thickness. T1 mapping before and 15 min after c.a. administration (0.1 mmol/kg). LGE images.

Main CMR Findings Left-ventricle volume and global function normal. Diffuse hypertrophy of ventricular wall (max 19 mm at the level of middle inferoseptal wall. Normal right ventricle. Abnormal thickness of right-ventricle free wall (Movie 1.29, Movie 1.30 and Movie 1.31).

Native T1 value: 835 ms within the myocardium not involved in the fibrotic process. Pseudo-normalization of T1 values in the regions of myocardium where LGE images show intramural fibrosis (1067 ms) at the level of the infero-lateral segments. ECV 24%.

Conclusion Anderson-Fabry disease.

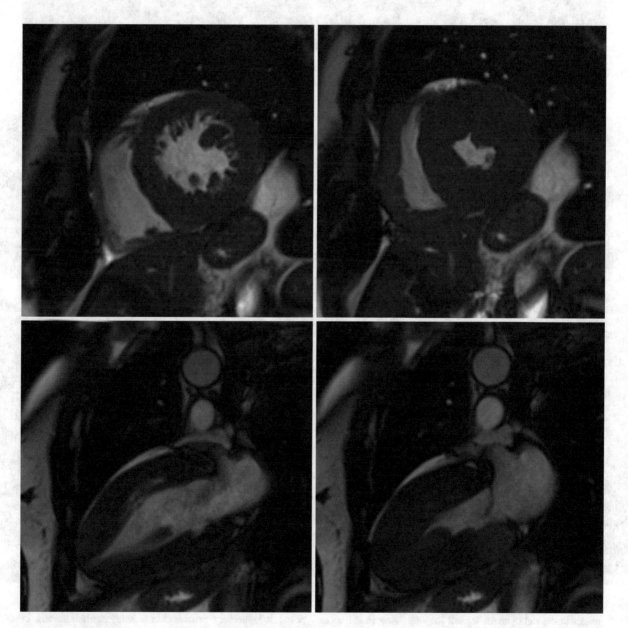

Fig. 1.36 SSFP cine images in short-axis (upper panels), vertical long-axis (middle panels), and horizontal long-axis (lower panels) views. Segmental hypertrophy in the presence of normal function. Left panels: diastolic frames; right panels: systolic frames

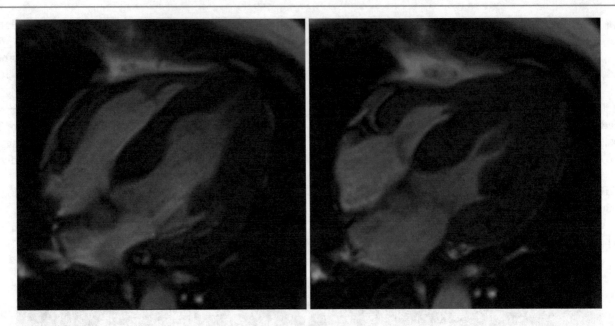

Fig. 1.36 (continued)

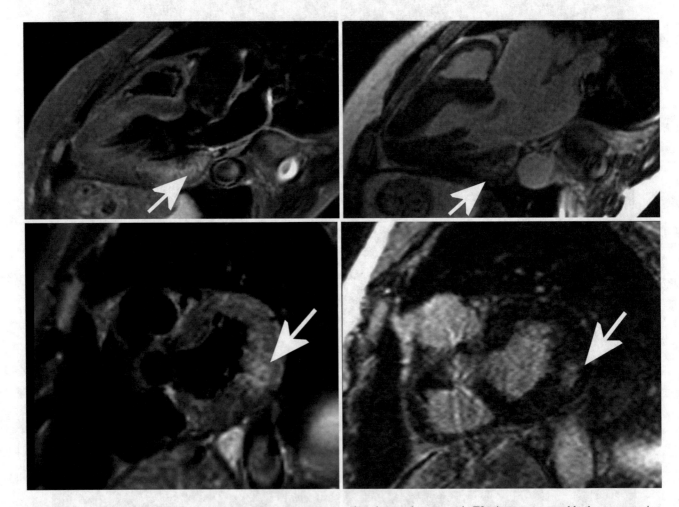

Fig. 1.37 T2-weighted images in the left panels and the correspondent LGE images in the right panels. Vertical long-axis view in the upper panels. Short-axis views in the middle and lower panels. The arrows show hyperenhancement in T2w images presumably due to a superimposed inflammatory process and intramyocardial fibrosis in LGE images

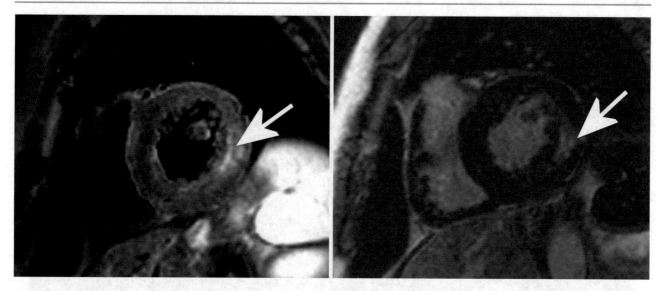

Fig. 1.37 (continued)

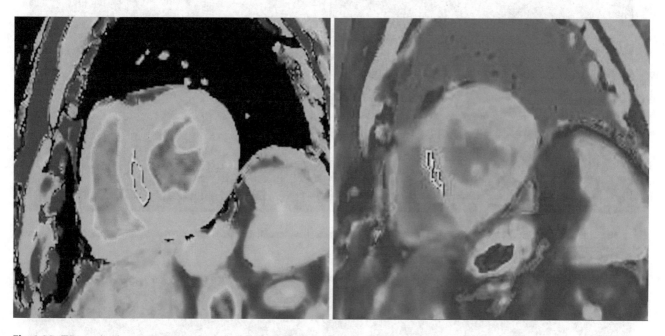

Fig. 1.38 T1 mapping images in short-axis view of the heart. Left panel: native T1 map, postcontrast T1 map

1.6.2   Cardiac Amyloidosis with Asymmetric Pseudohypertrophy

Medical History Male, 63 y.o. Hypertension. Multiple myeloma. Annual follow-up.

CMR Flowchart Stack of cine images in short-axis view to evaluate biventricular volumes and function. T1 mapping (sh-MOLLI) before and after administration of a bolus of contrast agent (0.1 mmol/kg). LGE images 10 min after the injection of c.a.

Main CMR Findings Normal regional and global left ventricular function. Asymmetric hypertrophy (16 mm at the level of the middle inferoseptal segment (16 mm)) (Movie 1.32, Movie 1.33 and Movie 1.34). Postcontrast LGE images show a diffuse uptake of contrast agent with a subendocardial pattern. Native T1 value = 1050 ± 26 ms (normal value, Piechnik et al.: 962 ± 25 ms JCMR 2013; ECV 42% (normal value 25 ± 3%)) (Fontana et al. JCMR 2012).

Conclusion Amyloidosis with involvement of the heart. Presence of of asymmetric pseudohypertrophy.

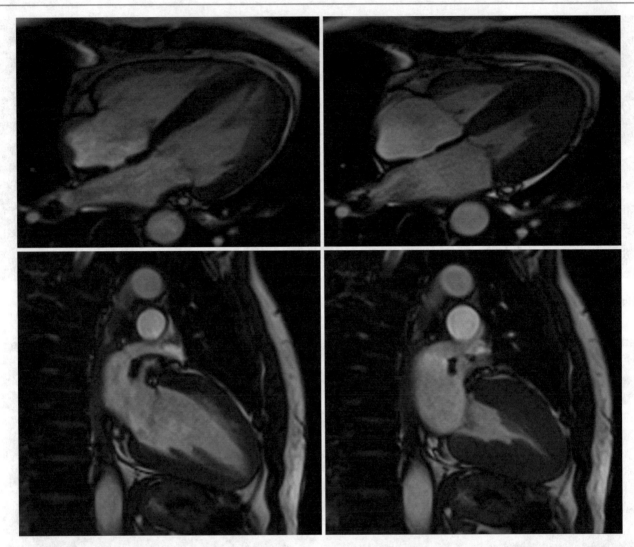

Fig. 1.39 Cine SSFP images showing asymmetric hypertrophy. Upper panels: horizontal long axis. Lower panels: vertical long axis. Left panels: end-diastolic phase. Right panels: end-systolic phase

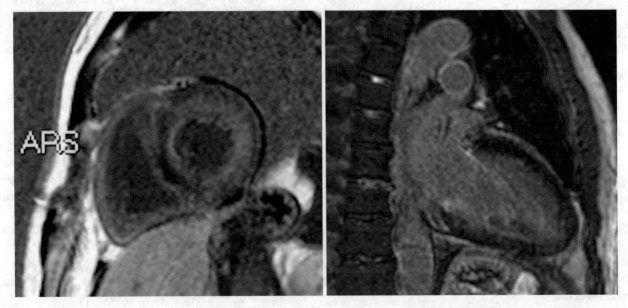

Fig. 1.40 LGE images. Left upper panel: short axis view, early acquisition after-contrast agent administration. Right upper panel: late acquisition in vertical long axis. Lower left panel: Late acquisition in short-axis view. Right lower panel: late acquisition in three-chamber view. In all images evidence of diffuse subendocardial uptake of the contrast agent

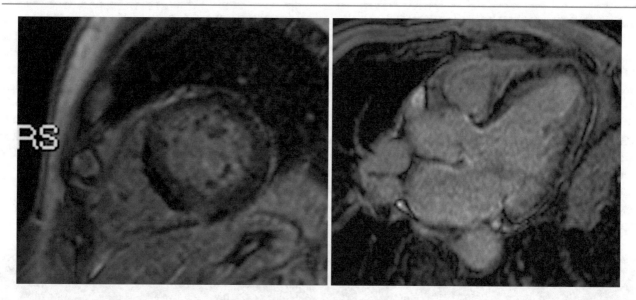

Fig. 1.40 (continued)

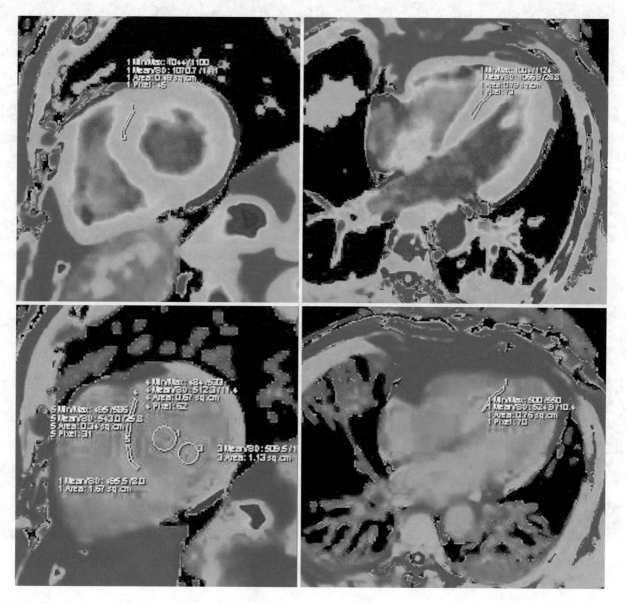

Fig. 1.41 T1 mapping pre- (upper panels) and postcontrast agent (lower panels) in short-axis view (left panel) and in horizontal long-axis view (right panel)

1.6.3   Cardiac Amyloidosis with Diffuse Pseudohypertrophy

Medical History   Male, 70 y.o. Since 1 year echocardiographic diagnosis of cardiac hypertrophy, EF 40%, pattern of diastolic impairment.

CMR Flowchart   Stack of cine images in short-axis view to evaluate biventricular volumes, regional and global function, and segmental thickness. Images in T2w and LGE (PSIR) for tissue characterization. T1 mapping images before contrast agent to evaluate native myocardial T1 and postcontrast agent (0.1 mmol/kg) to evaluate ECV.

Main CMR Findings   Left-ventricle volume within normal limits with reduction of global function (EF 36%). Diffuse myocardial hypertrophy (max thickness at the level of septal segments: 19 mm). Increased myocardial mass (153 g/m^2). The pseudohypertrophic process involves the right-ventricle free wall (average thickness: 7 mm) (Movie 1.35 and Movie 1.36). Increased native T1 values. Diffuse subendocardial c.a. uptake in LGE images with evidence of a marked hypointense signal of the blood and severely increased ECV (>50%).

Conclusion   Amyloidosis with diffuse pseudohypertrophy and impairment of global left ventricular function.

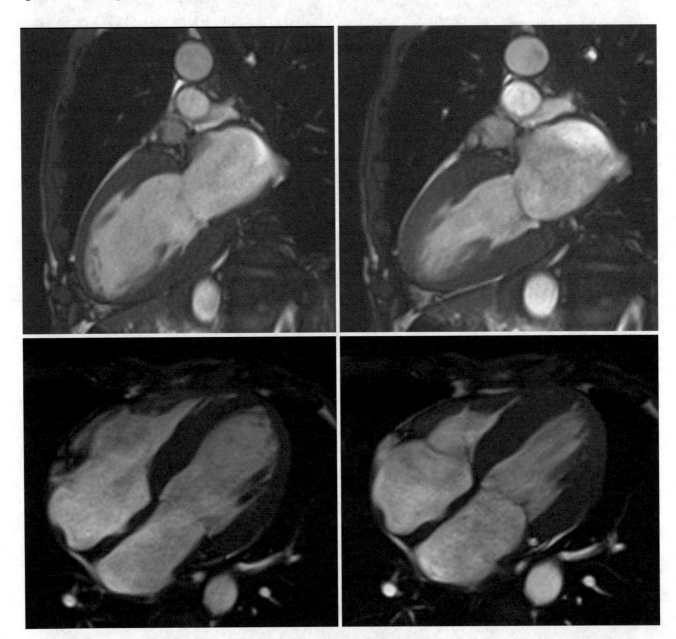

Fig. 1.42   SSFP cine images in vertical (upper panels) and horizontal (lower panels) planes. Evidence of myocardial hypertrophy involving also the right-ventricle free wall. Left panels: diastolic frames. Right panels: systolic frames

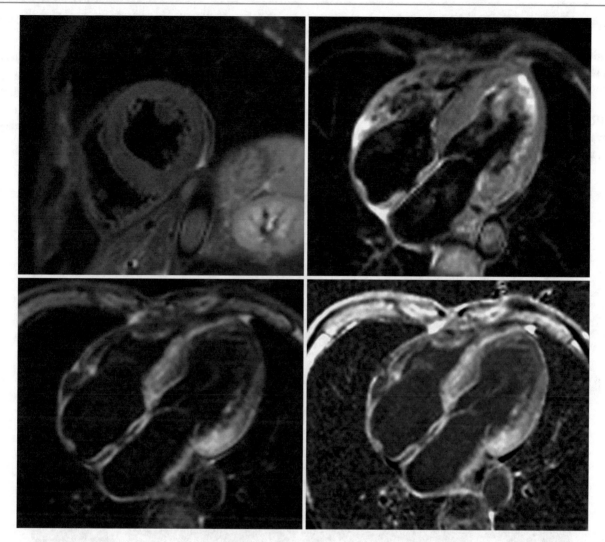

Fig. 1.43 T2-weighted images (upper panels) in short axis (left) and horizontal long axis (right). No evidence of myocardial signal abnormalities. In phase-sensitive inversion recovery (PSIR) reconstruction (lower panels) diffuse uptake of the contrast agent (subendocardial or almost transmural) and evidence of a persistent marked hypointense signal from the blood, which appears indeed black. Lower left panel: magnitude inversion recovery image. Lower right panel: phase-sensitive image

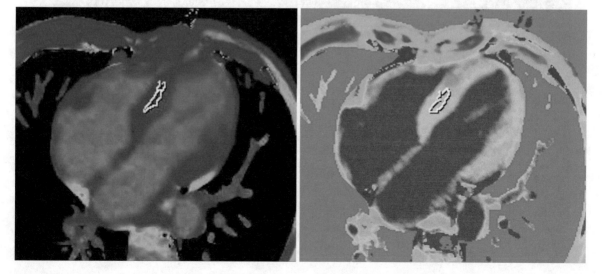

Fig. 1.44 Native T1 map of the myocardium (left panel) and postcontrast T1 map (right panel). The native T1 measured within the region of interest at the level of the interventricular septum resulted in 1120 ms and 358 ms 15 min after the administration of contrast agent (0.1 mmol/kg). The calculated ECV >50%

1.6.4   Glycogen Storage Disease

Medical History Male, 21 y.o. Genetically proven glycogen storage disease. Evidence of myocardial hypertrophy at Echocardiography.

CMR Flowchart Stack of cine images in short-axis view to evaluate biventricular volumes, regional and global function, and segmental thickness. Stack of T2w images in short axis and vertical and horizontal long axis to assess the presence of myocardial edema. LGE images to detect myocardial fibrosis.

Main CMR Findings Diffuse hypertrophy, more evident at the level of the interventricular septum (27 mm) (Movie 1.37, Movie 1.38 and Movie 1.39). Turbulence of flow at the level of the outflow tract. Multiple areas of signal abnormalities in T2w images. Multiple areas of contrast agent uptake in LGE images.

Conclusion Myocardial involvement in glycogen storage disease.

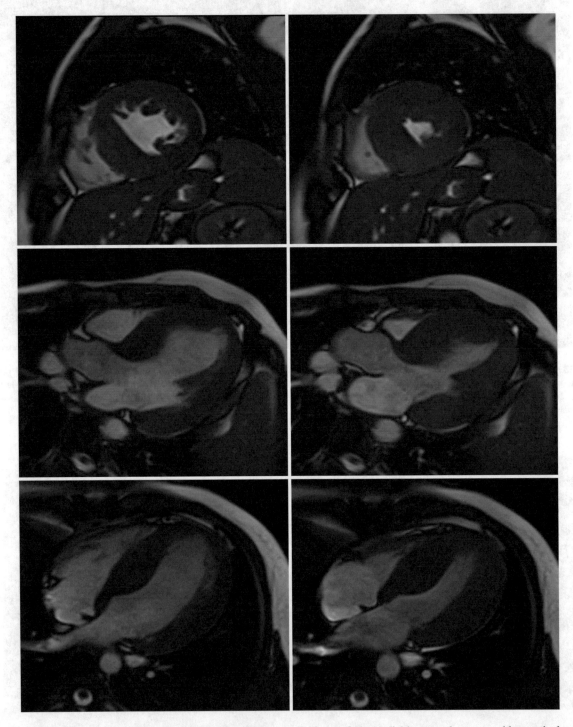

Fig. 1.45 SSFP cine images in short-axis view (upper panels), three-chamber view (middle panels), horizontal long-axis view (lower panels). Left panels: end-diastolic frames, right panels: end-systolic frames. Evidence of myocardial hypertrophy, more evident at the level of the interventricular septum

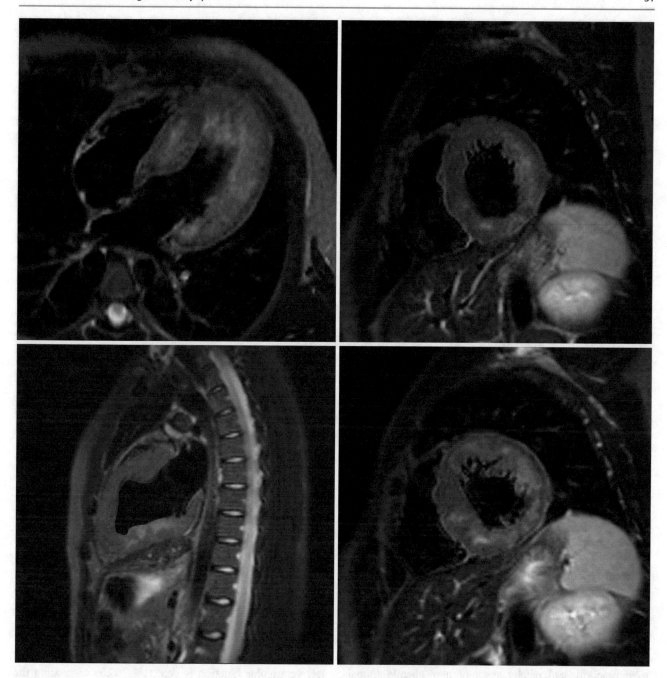

Fig. 1.46 T2w images. Upper left panel: horizontal long axis. Lower left panel: vertical long axis. Right panels: two parallel short-axis views of the heart

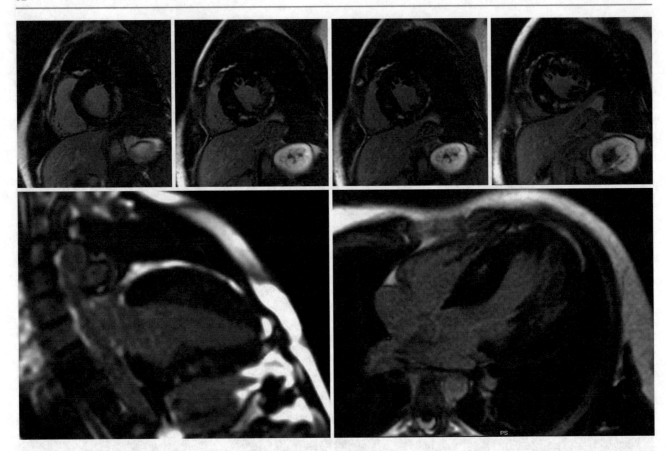

Fig. 1.47 LGE images. Upper panels: four parallel short-axis views of the heart. Lower left panel: vertical long axis. Lower right panel: horizontal long axis. Evidence of multiple areas of contrast uptake

1.6.5 Iron Overload Cardiomyopathy

Medical History Male, 27 y.o. In 2008, affected by Thalassemia major. Regular monthly transfusion therapy since 1 year of age. Chelated with deferoxamine since he was 3 y.o. In 2008 underwent the first CMR study with evidence of severe and homogeneous cardiac iron overload, a borderline liver iron burden, a mild depression of global systolic function, and patchy areas of nonischemic fibrosis. Based on the CMR findings a combined chelation therapy (deferiprone and deferoxamine) was started.

In 2012 the patient underwent a second CMR study with evidence of a significant reduction in the cardiac iron burden showing a heterogeneous myocardial iron overload, no liver iron burden, and a normalization of the global systolic function. In 2014 a further CMR study showed no evidence of liver and myocardial iron overload in any segment with a normal left global systolic function; the patchy areas of nonischemic fibrosis showed no progression since 2008. So, the intensive combined chelation therapy was stopped and the oral deferiprone in monotherapy was continued.

CMR Flowchart Stack of cine images in short-axis view to evaluate biventricular volumes and function. T2* images of the heart in short-axis view. LGE images.

Main CMR Findings A progressive improvement of global left ventricular function is detectable when comparing the results of the first (Movie 1.40), the second and the third (Movie 1.41) CMR study. Symmetrically, an increase of T2* values have been detected indicating a progressive reduction of iron burden.

Conclusion A segmental T2* CMR (Meloni et al. EHJ CVI 2015) permits a strictly tailored patient chelation therapy, leading to a lower risk of iron-mediated heart failure and of arrhythmias than previously reported (Pepe et al. EHJ CVI 2018).

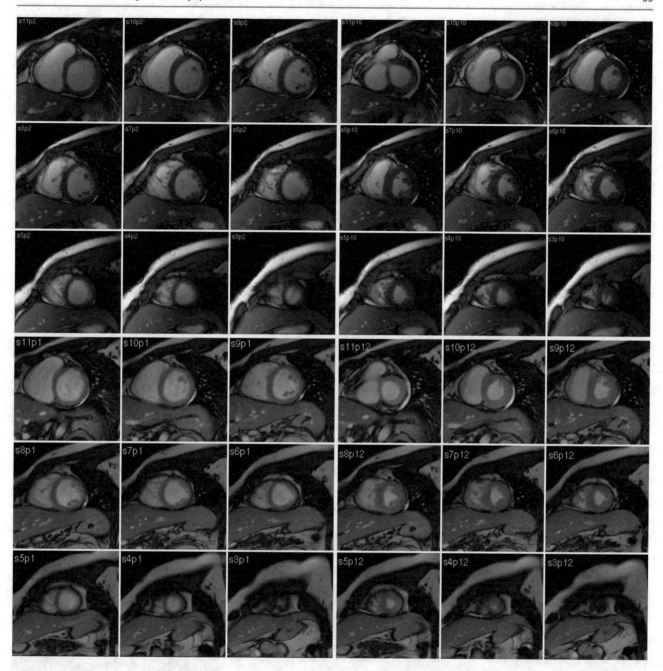

Fig. 1.48 Stack of SSFP cine images in nine short axis covering the whole heart, before (upper three rows) and after 6 years (lower three rows) of optimized chelation therapy. Left three columns: diastolic frames. Right three columns: systolic frames. Evidence of improved global function of left ventricle

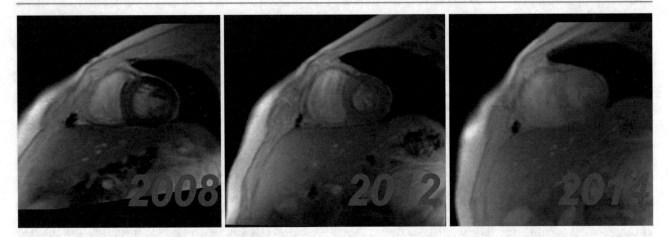

Fig. 1.49 T2* GRE multiecho images (TE 4.4) in short-axis view of left ventricle. Evidence of a progressive signal intensity increase on the years at the level of the heart and at the level of the liver

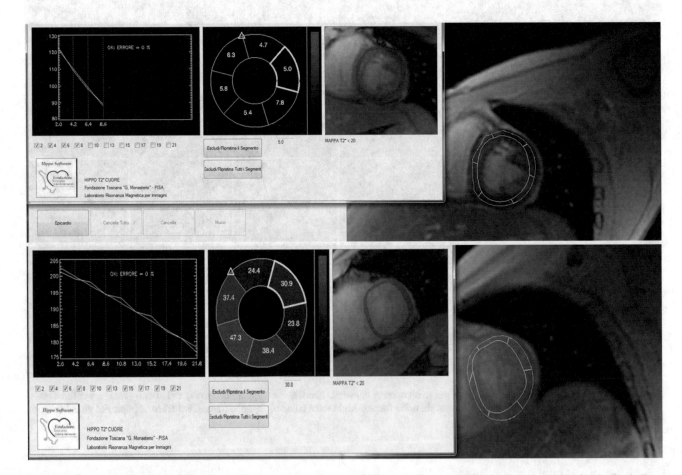

Fig. 1.50 Analysis of T2* GRE images by a segmental approach using a previously validated software (HIPPO MIOT) (Pepe et al. JMRI 2006). Upper panel: images obtained before optimizing the chelation therapy based on MR. The myocardial signal decay on time is very fast indicating a severe iron overload. In the lower panel a significant improvement is evidenced by a substantial slowdown of signal decay on time

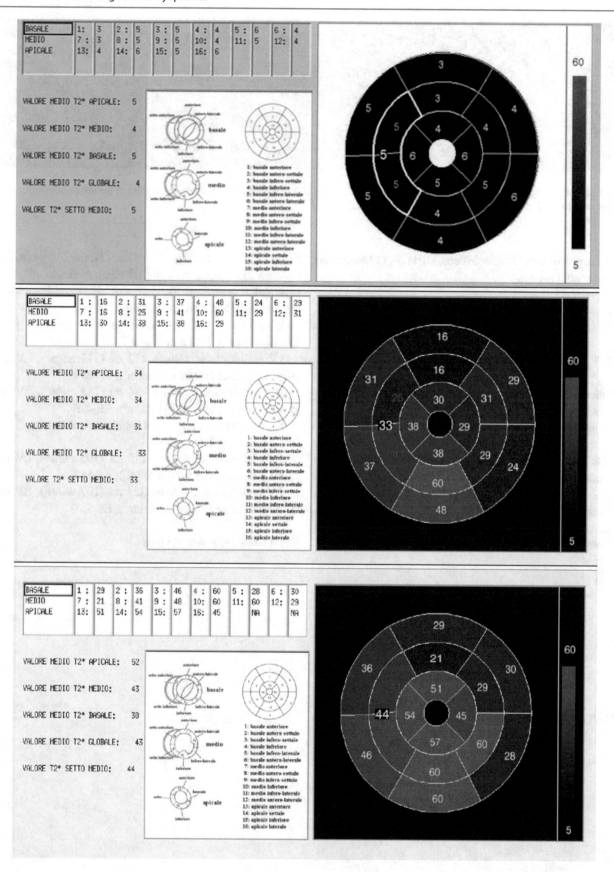

Fig. 1.51 Analysis of T2* mapping by a segmental approach using a previously validated software (HIPPO MIOT). Upper panel: a homogeneous iron overload is present leading to a diffuse pathological reduction of T2* in all segments (<20 ms). In the middle panel a significant improvement is obtained after the optimization of the chelation therapy with a heterogenous myocardial iron overload and a global heart T2* value >20 ms; only few segments still show a pathological reduction in T2* values (<20 ms). In the lower panel a complete normalization of T2* values in all segments (>20 ms) is detected indicating the success of chelation therapy

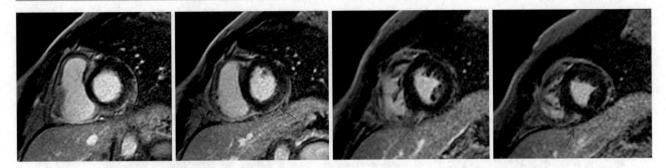

Fig. 1.52 LGE images obtained after the administration of gadobutrol (0.2 mmol/kg). Evidence of enhancement at the level of the basal infero-lateral wall, the mid- and distal inferior septal junction (arrows)

Case provided by Dr. Alessia Pepe, MRI Lab, G. Monasterio Foundation, Pisa, Italy.

1.7 Adaptive Cardiomyopathies

1.7.1 Athlete Heart

Medical History Male, 21 y.o. Asymptomatic. Heavy sportsman (professional biker).

Dilatation of both ventricles at Echocardiography.

CMR Flowchart Stack of cine images in short-axis view to evaluate biventricular volumes and function. Stack of images in short axis of the heart in black blood weighted in Proton Density and in LGE to exclude the possibility of morpho-structural abnormalities. Same images obtained baseline and 6 months after a complete stop of sport physical activity.

Main CMR Findings Baseline: Normal biventricular regional and global function. Normal thickness of all the myocardial segments. No structural abnormalities. Normal dimension of both the left and right atrium.

Dilatation of both the ventricles with preserved global function (Movie 1.42 and Movie 1.44).

LV end-diastolic volume 242 ml (117 ml/m^2), LV end-systolic volume 109 ml (53 ml/m^2); EF 55%.

RV end-diastolic volume 298 ml (143 ml/m^2), RV end-systolic volume 168 ml (81 ml/m^2); EF 45%.

Six months after the stop of sport physical activity (Movie 1.43 and Movie 1.45).

LV end-diastolic volume 219 ml (105 ml/m^2), LV end-systolic volume 101 ml (48 ml/m^2); EF 54%.

RV end-diastolic volume 224 ml (107 ml/m^2), RV end-systolic volume 105 ml (50 ml/m^2); EF 53%.

Final Diagnosis Athlete heart.

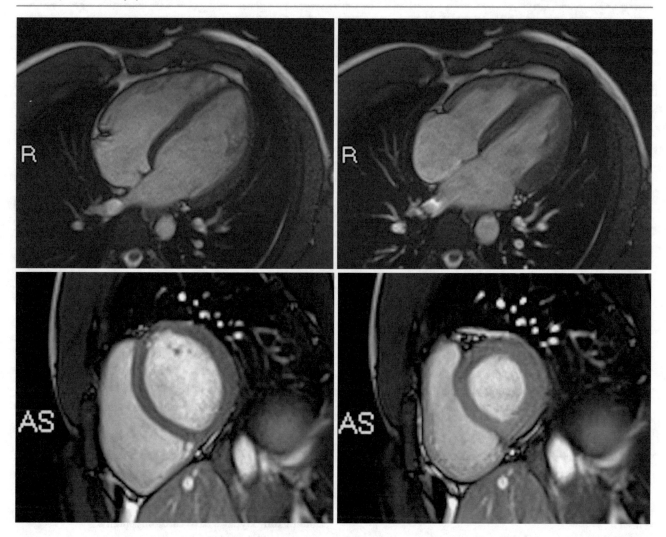

Fig. 1.53 Stack of SSFP cine images in horizontal long-axis (upper panels) and in short-axis view (lower panels) of the heart. End-diastolic frames (left panels) and end-systolic frames (right panels). Images collected at baseline

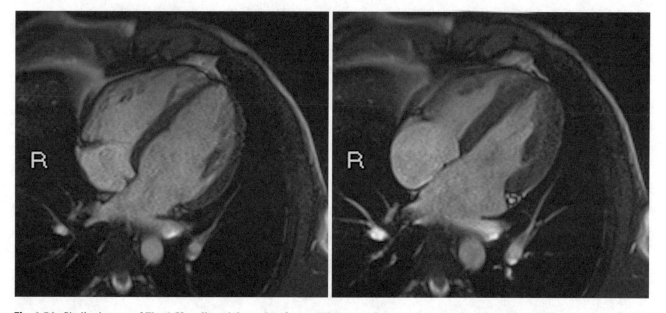

Fig. 1.54 Similar images of Fig. 1.53, collected 6 months after complete stop of sport activity. At visual inspection no changes are detectable. However the quantitative measurement of volumes clearly shows a significant reduction of volumes of both ventricles

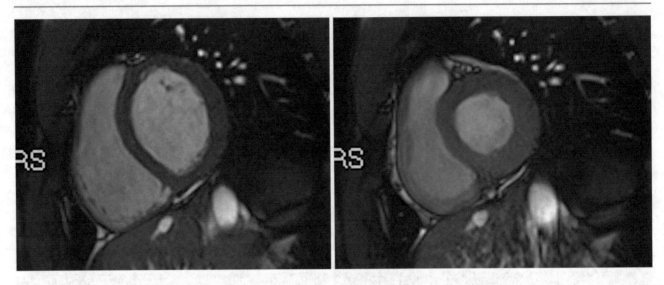

Fig. 1.54 (continued)

1.7.2 Hypertensive Cardiomyopathy

Medical History 56-year-old woman patient with a history of arterial hypertension. Microcythemia trait. Hypertrophy of the left ventricle at Echocardiography. Diagnostic suspect of amyloidosis.

MR Flow Chart Stack of cine images in short-axis view to evaluate biventricular volumes and function. Stack of T2w and LGE images in short-axis view of left ventricle for tissue characterization.

Main CMR Findings Normal sizes, volumes, and function of the left ventricle. Hypertrophy of the left ventricle more signed in the anterior and anteroseptal wall in the mid-basal segments (max thickness at the level of the basal anteroseptal segment: 14 mm). Increase of myocardial mass (100 g/m^2) (n.v. $47–77 \text{ g/m}^2$) (Movie 1.46 and Movie 1.47).

Normal range of sizes, volumes, and function of the ventricle.

No signs of edema or fibrosis in the myocardium.

Unexpected CMR finding: right-sided aortic arch with a course of the thoracic Aorta to the right of the spine (see Chap. 7).

Conclusion Hypertensive cardiomyopathy.

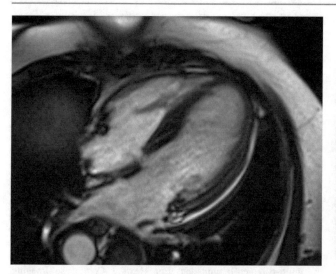

Fig. 1.55 End-diastolic frame from a SSFP cine sequence. Horizontal long axis. Evidence of light hypertrophy at the level of proximal septal segment

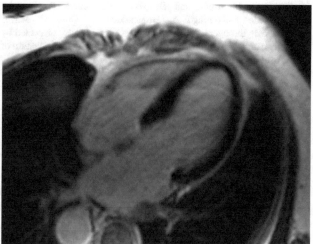

Fig. 1.57 LGE image in horizontal long axis. No uptake of c.a.

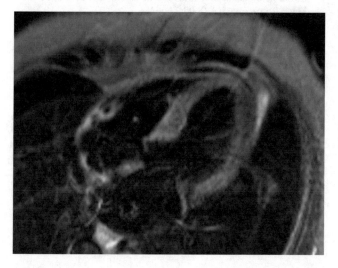

Fig. 1.56 T2w image in horizontal long axis. No signal abnormalities

Bibliography

1. Maron MS, Maron BJ. Clinical impact of contemporary cardiovascular magnetic resonance imaging in hypertrophic cardiomyopathy. Circulation. 2015;132(4):292–8.
2. Chan C, Maron MS. Hypertrophic cardiomyopathy. The EACVI textbook of cardiovascular magnetic resonance: Oxford University Press; 2018.
3. Maron MS, Olivotto I, Maron BJ, Prasad SK, Cecchi F, Udelson JE, Camici PG. The case for myocardial ischemia in hypertrophic cardiomyopathy. J Am Coll Cardiol. 2009;54(9):866–75.
4. Haaf P, Garg P, Messroghli DR, Broadbent DA, Greenwood JP, Plein S. Cardiac T1 mapping and extracellular volume (ECV) in clinical practice: a comprehensive review. J Cardiovasc Magn Reson. 2016;18(1):89.
5. Gulati A, Ismail TF, Prasad SK. Fibrosis and mortality in patients with dilated cardiomyopathy—reply. JAMA. 2013;309(24):2548–9.
6. Gulati A, Jabbour A, Ismail TF, Guha K, Khwaja J, Raza S, Morarji K, Brown TD, Ismail NA, Dweck MR, Di Pietro E, Roughton M, Wage R, Daryani Y, O'Hanlon R, Sheppard MN, Alpendurada F, Lyon AR, Cook SA, Cowie MR, Assomull RG, Pennell DJ, Prasad SK. Association of fibrosis with mortality and sudden cardiac death in patients with nonischemic dilated cardiomyopathy. JAMA. 2013;309(9):896–908.
7. Dweck MR, Joshi S, Murigu T, Alpendurada F, Jabbour A, Melina G, Banya W, Gulati A, Roussin I, Raza S, Prasad NA, Wage R, Quarto C, Angeloni E, Refice S, Sheppard M, Cook SA, Kilner PJ, Pennell DJ, Newby DE, Mohiaddin RH, Pepper J, Prasad SK. Midwall fibrosis is an independent predictor of mortality in patients with aortic stenosis. J Am Coll Cardiol. 2011;58(12):1271–9.
8. Lombardi M, Plein S, Petersen S, Bucciarelli-Ducci C, Valsangiacomo-Buechel M, Basso C, Ferrari V. The EACVI Textbook of Cardiovascular Magnetic Resonance. Oxford; Oxford University Press; 2018.
9. Petersen SE, Selvanayagam JB, Wiesmann F, Robson MD, Francis JM, Anderson RH, Watkins H, Neubauer S. Left ventricular non-compaction: insights from cardiovascular magnetic resonance imaging. J Am Coll Cardiol. 2005;46(1):101–5.
10. Jacquier A, Thuny F, Jop B, Giorgi R, Cohen F, Gaubert JY, Vidal V, Bartoli JM, Habib G, Moulin G. Measurement of trabeculated left ventricular mass using cardiac magnetic resonance imaging in the diagnosis of left ventricular non-compaction. Eur Heart J. 2010;31(9):1098–104.
11. Aquaro GD, Pingitore A, Strata E, Di Bella G, Molinaro S, Lombardi M. Cardiac magnetic resonance predicts outcome in patients with premature ventricular complexes of left bundle branch block morphology. J Am Coll Cardiol. 2010;56(15):1235–43.
12. Marra MP, Leoni L, Bauce B, Corbetti F, Zorzi A, Migliore F, Silvano M, Rigato I, Tona F, Tarantini G, Cacciavillani L, Basso C, Buja G, Thiene G, Iliceto S, Corrado D. Imaging study of ventricular scar in arrhythmogenic right ventricular cardiomyopathy: comparison of 3D standard electroanatomical voltage mapping and contrast-enhanced cardiac magnetic resonance. Circ Arrhythm Electrophysiol. 2012;5(1):91–100.
13. Rastegar N, Zimmerman SL, Te Riele ASJM, James C, Burt JR, Bhonsale A, Murray B, Tichnell C, Judge D, Calkins H, Tandri H, Bluemke DA, Kamel IR. Spectrum of Biventricular Involvement on CMR Among Carriers of ARVD/C-Associated Mutations. JACC Cardiovasc Imaging. 2015;8(7):863–4.

14. Saguner AM, Buchmann B, Wyler D, Manka R, Gotschy A, Medeiros-Domingo A, Brunckhorst C, Duru F, Mayer KA. Arrhythmogenic left ventricular cardiomyopathy suspected by cardiac magnetic resonance imaging, confirmed by identification of a novel plakophilin-2 variant. Circulation. 2015;132:e38–40.

15. Bennett RG, Haqqani HM, Berruezo A, Della Bella P, Marchlinski FE, Hsu CJ, Kumar S. Arrhythmogenic Cardiomyopathy in 2018-2019: ARVC/ALVC or Both? Heart Lung Circ. 2019;28(1):164–77.

16. Weidemann F, Rummey C, Bijnens B, Störk S, Jasaityte R, Dhooge J, Baltabaeva A, Sutherland G, Schulz JB, Meier T. The heart in Friedreich ataxia: definition of cardiomyopathy, disease severity, and correlation with neurological symptoms. Circulation. 2012;125(13):1626–34.

17. Meyer C, Schmid G, Görlitz S, Ernst M, Wilkens C, Wilhelms I, Kraus PH, Bauer P, Tomiuk J, Przuntek H, Mügge A, Schöls L. Cardiomyopathy in Friedreich's ataxia-assessment by cardiac MRI. Mov Disord. 2007;22(11):1615–22.

18. Schmacht L, Traber J, Grieben U, Utz W, Dieringer MA, Kellman P, Blaszczyk E, von Knobelsdorff-Brenkenhoff F, Spuler S, Schulz-Menger J. Cardiac involvement in myotonic dystrophy type 2 patients with preserved ejection fraction: detection by cardiovascular magnetic resonance. Circ Cardiovasc Imaging. 2016;9(7).

19. Turkbey EB, Gai N, Lima JA, van der Geest RJ, Wagner KR, Tomaselli GF, Bluemke DA, Nazarian S. Assessment of cardiac involvement in myotonic muscular dystrophy by T1 mapping on magnetic resonance imaging. Heart Rhythm. 2012;9(10):1691–7.

20. Verhaert D, Richards K, Rafael-Fortney JA, Raman SV. Cardiac involvement in patients with muscular dystrophies magnetic resonance imaging phenotype and genotypic considerations. Circ Cardiovasc Imaging. 2011;4:67–76.

21. Camporeale A, Pieroni M, Pieruzzi F, Lusardi P, Pica S, Spada M, Mignani R, Burlina A, Bandera F, Guazzi M, Graziani F, Crea F, Greiser A, Boveri S, Ambrogi F, Lombardi M. Predictors of clinical evolution in prehypertrophic Fabry disease. Circ Cardiovasc Imaging. 2019;12(4):e008424.

22. Fontana M, Pica S, Reant P, Abdel-Gadir A, Treibel TA, Banypersad SM, Maestrini V, Barcella W, Rosmini S, Bulluck H, Sayed RH, Patel K, Mamhood S, Bucciarelli-Ducci C, Whelan CJ, Herrey AS, Lachmann HJ, Wechalekar AD, Manisty CH, Schelbert EB, Kellman P, Gillmore JD, Hawkins PN, Moon JC. Prognostic value of late gadolinium enhancement cardiovascular magnetic resonance in cardiac amyloidosis. Circulation. 2015;132(16):1570–9.

23. Fontana M, Banypersad SM, Treibel TA, Maestrini V, Sado DM, White SK, Pica S, Castelletti S, Piechnik SK, Robson MD, Gilbertson JA, Rowczenio D, Hutt DF, Lachmann HJ, Wechalekar AD, Whelan CJ, Gillmore JD, Hawkins PN, Moon JC. Native T1 mapping in transthyretin amyloidosis. JACC Cardiovasc Imaging. 2014;7(2):157–65.

24. Meloni A, Positano V, Ruffo GB, Spasiano A, D'Ascola D, Peluso A, Petra K, Gennaro R, Valeri G, Renne S, Midiri M, Pepe A. Improvement of heart iron with preserved patterns of iron store by CMR-guided chelation therapy. Eur Heart J Cardiovasc Imaging. 2015;16(3):325–34.

25. Pepe A, Meloni A, Rossi G, Midiri M, Missere M, Valeri G, Sorrentino F, D'Ascola DG, Spasiano A, Filosa A, Cuccia L, Dello Iacono N, Forni G, Caruso V, Maggio A, Pitrolo L, Peluso A, De Marchi D, Positano V, Wood JC. Prediction of cardiac complications for thalassemia major in the widespread cardiac magnetic resonance era: a prospective multicentre study by a multi-parametric approach. Eur Heart J Cardiovasc Imaging. 2018;19(3):299–309.

26. Pepe A, Positano V, Santarelli MF, Sorrentino F, Cracolici E, De Marchi D, Maggio A, Midiri M, Landini L, Lombardi M. Multislice multiecho T2* Cardiovascular Magnetic Resonance for detection of the heterogeneous distribution of myocardial iron overload. J Magn Reson Imaging. 2006;23:662–8.

27. D'Ascenzi F, Anselmi F, Piu P, Fiorentini C, Carbone SF, Volterrani L, Focardi M, Bonifazi M, Mondillo S. Cardiac magnetic resonance normal reference values of biventricular size and function in male athlete's heart. JACC Cardiovasc Imaging. 2018.

28. Petersen SE, Selvanayagam JB, Francis JM, Myerson SG, Wiesmann F, Robson MD, Ostman-Smith I, Casadei B, Watkins H, Neubauer S. Differentiation of athlete's heart from pathological forms of cardiac hypertrophy by means of geometric indices derived from cardiovascular magnetic resonance. J Cardiovasc Magn Reson. 2005;7(3):551–8.

29. EACVI textbook of cardiovascular magnetic resonance. Oxford University Press; 2018.

30. Karam R, Lever HM. Healy BP. Hypertensive hypertrophic cardiomyopathy or hypertrophic cardiomyopathy with hypertension? A study of 78 patients. J Am Coll Cardiol. 1989;13(3):580–4.

Myocarditis

2.1 Acute Inflammatory Processes

2.1.1 Acute Myocarditis

Clinical History 26-year-old male patient with history of hypertrophic myocardium.

In 2012 hospitalized for episode of myopericarditis. In March 2018 recurrence of chest pain and clinical diagnosis of myocarditis, treated with anti-inflammation drugs.

CMR Flowchart Stack of cine images in short-axis view to evaluate biventricular volumes and function. T2w images in horizontal and vertical long-axis and short-axis views (TR >1500 ms, TE >60 ms) to detect myocardial edema. Postcontrast LGE images to detect myocardial uptake.

Main CMR Findings Sizes and volumes of both ventricles are within normal range with normal biventricular systolic function (Movie 2.1 and Movie 2.2).

Presence of multiple areas of increased enhancement in T2w images as a result of the presence of myocardial edema.

Presence of multiple areas of contrast agent uptake in LGE images as a result of interstitial space expansion and myocyte necrosis.

At follow-up no areas of abnormal signal in T2 images while the extension of contrast uptake in LGE images is reduced.

Conclusion Acute myocarditis with the presence of edema and contrast uptake during the acute phase. Disappearance of edema in the follow-up.

Electronic Supplementary Material The online version of this chapter (https://doi.org/10.1007/978-3-030-41830-4_2) contains supplementary material, which is available to authorized users.

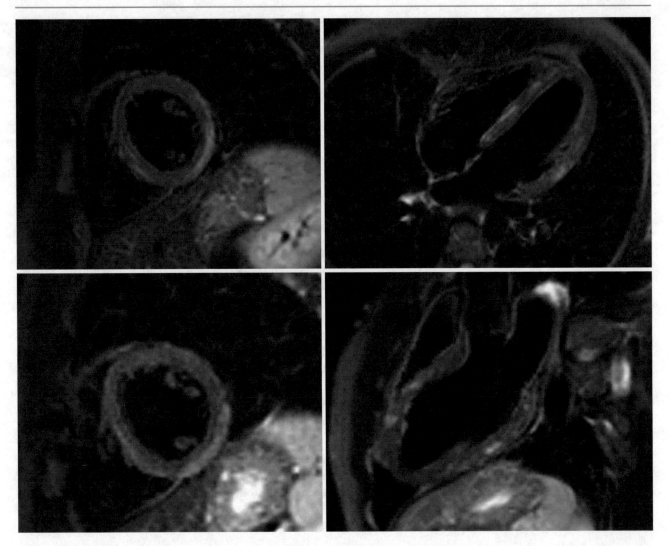

Fig. 2.1 T2w images in short axis (left upper and lower panel), horizontal long axis (right upper panel), and vertical long axis (right lower panel). Multiple areas of increased intensity within the myocardium indicating the presence of myocardial edema

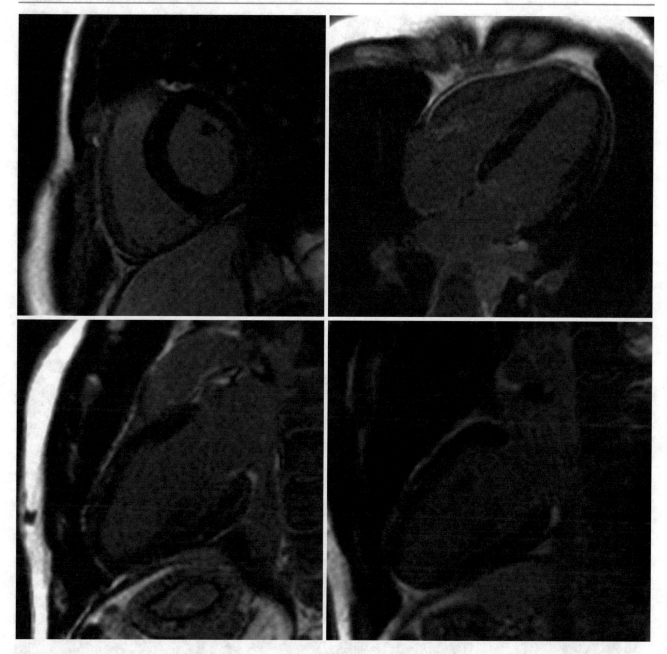

Fig. 2.2 Postcontrast LGE images in short axis (left upper panel), horizontal long axis (right upper panel), and two parallel vertical long axes of left ventricle (lower panels). Evidence of multiple areas of myocardial uptake of the contrast agent

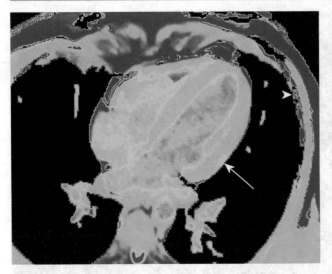

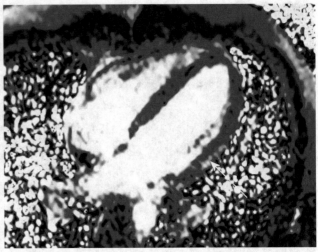

Fig. 2.3 T1 map of the myocardium during the acute phase of the disease. Horizontal long axis. The arrow shows the areas with longer native T1 values

Fig. 2.4 T2 map of the myocardium during the acute phase of the disease. Horizontal long axis. The arrow shows the areas with longer native T2 values

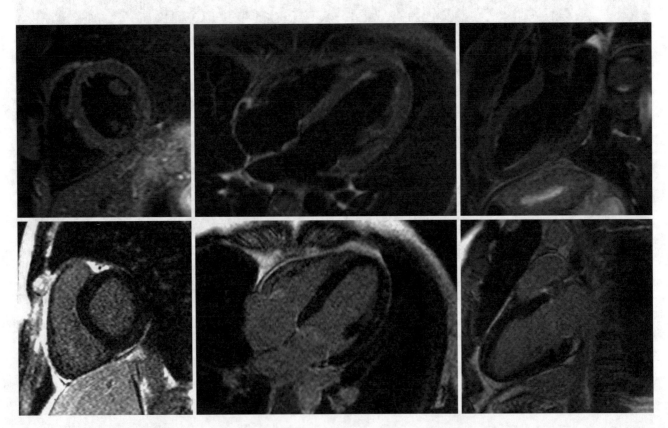

Fig. 2.5 T2w images (upper panels) and LGE images (lower panels) at follow-up. The disappearance of areas with abnormal signal is noticeable in T2 images, while the LGE images show still the uptake of con-trast agent but with a smaller extension and in a reduced number of areas when compared to the acute phase

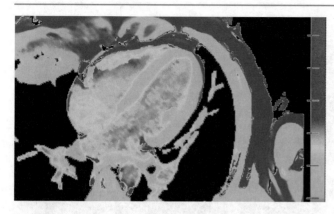

Fig. 2.6 T1 mapping image. There are no areas with abnormal/prolonged native T1 value

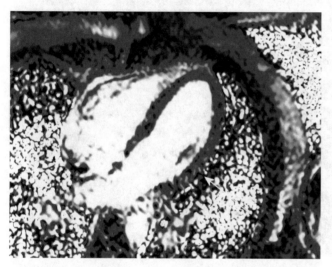

Fig. 2.7 T2 mapping image. There is a reduced extension of the area with abnormal T2 value (arrow) when compared with the same image obtained in the acute phase (Fig. 2.4)

2.1.2 Takotsubo Syndrome

Medical History Female, 57 y.o. Recent access to the emergency room because high fever, nausea, vomiting. marked reduction of the LV global function at Echocardiography. Rapid development of cardiogenic shock. No significant coronary stenosis.

CMR Flowchart Stack of cine images in short-axis view to evaluate biventricular volumes and function. Stack of cine images in vertical and horizontal long axis. T2w images in short and long axes. LGE images.

Main CMR Findings Severe regional and global function impairment with ballooning of the apical region of the heart (Movie 2.3 and Movie 2.4). Presence of diffuse increase of signal in T2w images in the apical regions. No contrast agent uptake in any segment of the myocardium.

Conclusion Takotsubo syndrome.

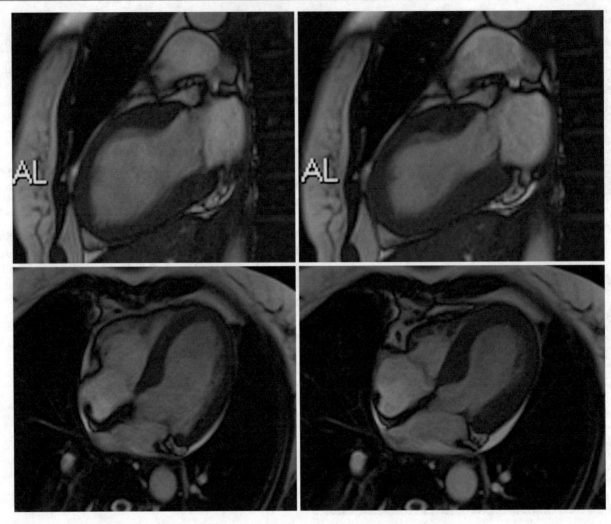

Fig. 2.8 SSFP cine images in vertical (upper panels) and in horizontal (lower panels). Evidence of apical ballooning during either the diastolic phase (left panels) or the systolic phase (right panels)

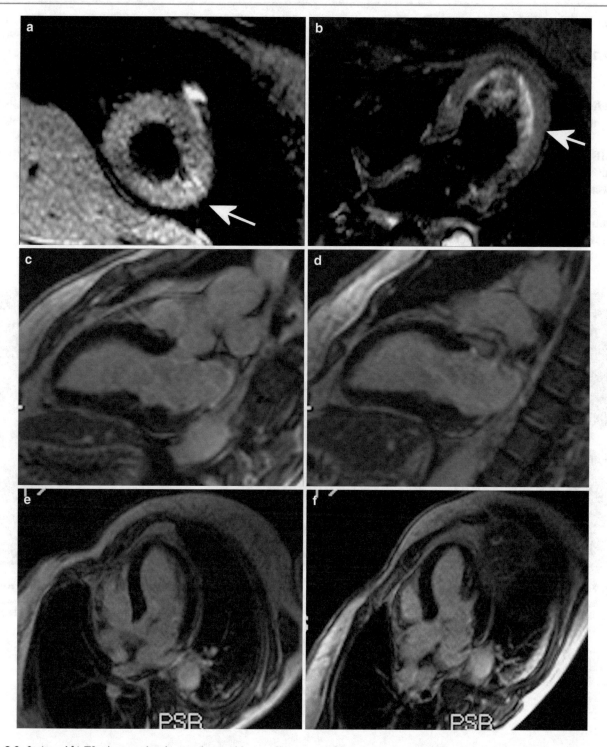

Fig. 2.9   In (**a** and **b**) T2w images showing an abnormal hyperenhancement of the myocardium at the level of the apical segments (arrows). In (**c**–**f**) LGE images in vertical and horizontal long axis with no evidence of myocardial uptake of c.a.

2.2 Chronic Inflammatory Processes

2.2.1 Chronic Myocarditis with Preserved Global Left Ventricular Function

Medical History Male, 16 y.o. Clinical and CMR-based diagnosis of acute myocarditis 3 years earlier. Asymptomatic.

CMR Flowchart Stack of cine images in short-axis view to evaluate biventricular volumes and function. T2w images to detect/exclude the presence of myocardial edema. LGE images.

Main CMR Findings During the acute phase: slight increase of left-ventricle volumes with preserved global function (EF 61%). No evidence of regional function abnormalities (Movie 2.5 and Movie 2.6). During the acute phase multiple signal abnormalities in SSFP cine images and in T2w images and multiple areas of c.a. uptake in LGE images, mainly at the level of lateral segments. At follow up evidence of preserved bi-venricular global and regional function (Movie 2.7 and Movie 2.8) no evidence of signal abnormalities both in SSFP images and in T2w images but clear evidence of contrast agent uptake in LGE images slightly reduced with respect to the acute phase.

Conclusion Chronic myocarditis. With preserved global left ventricular function.

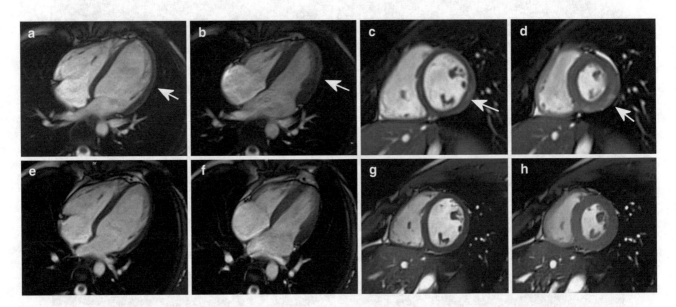

Fig. 2.10 SSFP cine images obtained during the acute phase (upper panels, in horizontal long-axis (a = diastole, b = systole) and in short-axis views (c = diastole, d = systole)) and after 3 years of follow-up (lower panels (e = diastole, f = systole) and in short-axis view (g = diastole, h = systole)). In the acute phase evidence (arrows) of diffuse pericardial/subepicardial hyperintensity which disappears in the follow-up

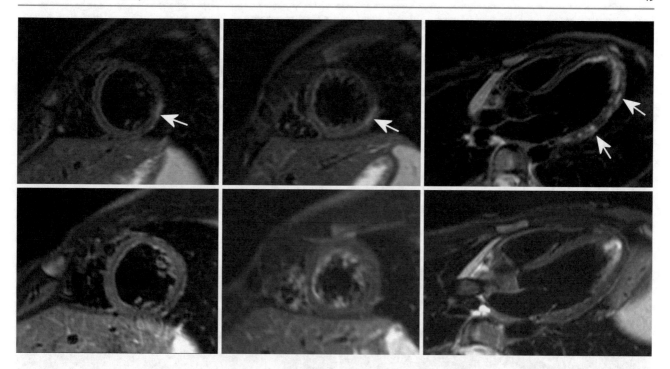

Fig. 2.11 T2-weighted images obtained during the acute phase (upper panels) in two short-axis views (left and middle panels) and in three-chamber view (right panel). In the lower panels the same images obtained 3 years later. The arrows show the presence, during the acute phase, of multiple areas of hyperintensity of the myocardium interpreted as due to myocardial edema

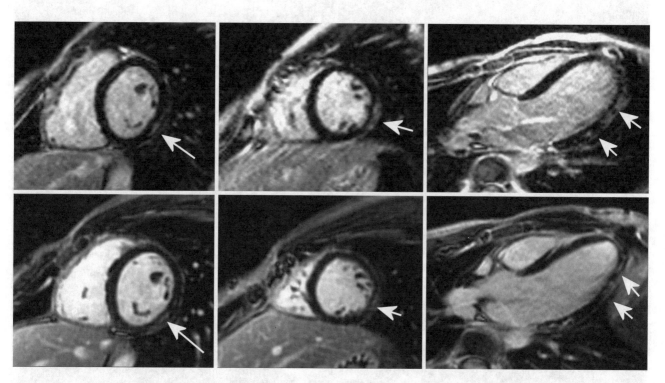

Fig. 2.12 LGE images obtained during the acute phase (upper panels) in two short-axis views (left and middle panels) and in three-chamber view (right panel). In the lower panels the same images obtained 3 years later. The arrows show the multiple areas of c.a. uptake at the level of the subepicardial layer and at the level of the pericardium

2.2.2   Chronic Myocarditis with Moderate Impairment of Global Left Ventricular Function

Medical History Male, 34 y.o. Previous diagnosis of non-specific cardiac arrhythmia. Episodes of pre-syncope. At Echocardiography slight reduction of global function and thickened pericardium.

CMR Flowchart Stack of cine images in short-axis view to evaluate biventricular volumes, function, and wall thickness. T2w images to detect/exclude the presence of myocardial edema. LGE images.

Main CMR Findings Light increase of left-ventricle volumes and reduction of global function (EF 48%). Evidence of diffuse hypokinesia (Movie 2.9, Movie 2.10 and Movie 2.11). No abnormalities in T2 images. Multiple areas of c.a. uptake in LGE images. Diffuse thickened pericardium. Pericardial effusion without any hemodynamic consequences.

Conclusion Chronic myopericarditis with moderate impairment of left ventricular global function. Pericardial thickening.

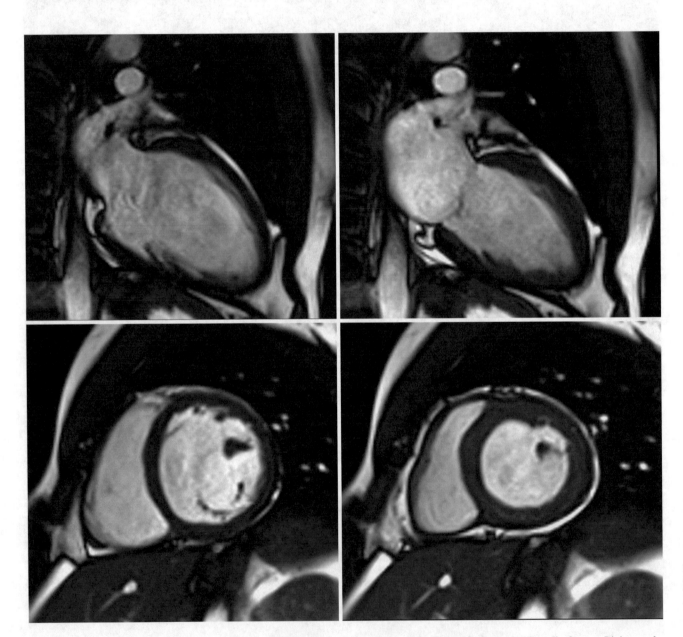

Fig. 2.13 SSFP cine images in vertical axis (upper panels) and in short-axis (lower panels) views. Evidence of slight increase of ventricular volumes and reduction of global function. Evidence of a nonsignifi-cant pericardial effusion. Left panels: diastolic frames. Right panels: systolic frames

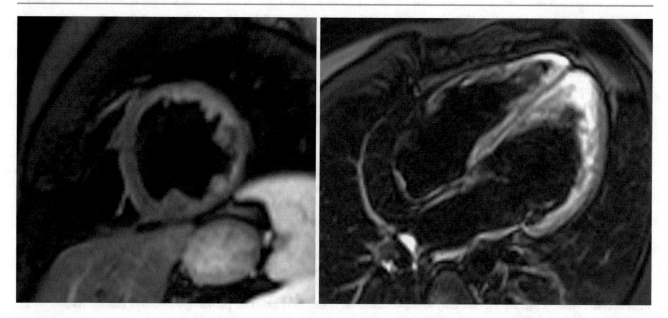

Fig. 2.14 T2-weighted images. Left panel: short-axis view. Right panel: horizontal long-axis view. No evidence of myocardial signal abnormalities

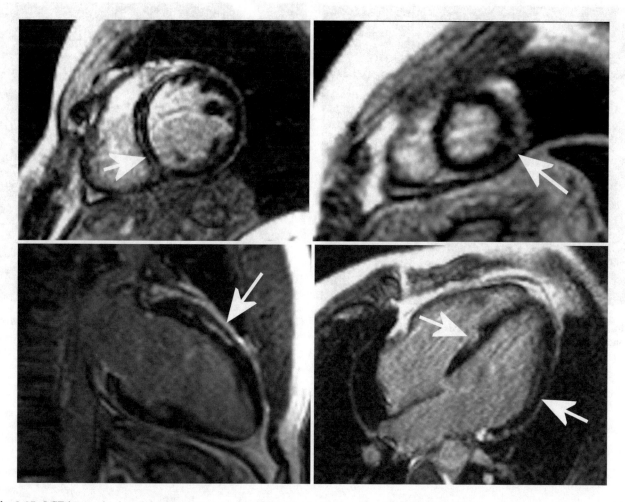

Fig. 2.15 LGE images in short-axis view (upper panels), vertical long-axis view (lower left panel), and horizontal long-axis view (lower right panel). The arrows show the multiple areas of c.a. uptake. There is also evidence of diffuse thickened pericardium

2.3   Post-chemo, Postradiation Cardiomyopathy

Medical History Female, 75 y.o. Family history of ischemic cardiac disease. On follow-up for breast cancer, treated by surgical intervention, and by chemo- and radiotherapy.

No major arrhythmia. Transthoracic Echocardiography showed dilatation of the left ventricle with diffusely reduced systolic function (LVEF: 42%), mild mitral regurgitation, and normal right heart diameters.

CMR Flowchart Stack of cine images in short axis to cover the whole-heart volume, for global and regional functional assessment; T2-weighted images to confirm/exclude the presence of myocardial edema; precontrast T1 mapping to assess native T1 values; LGE images to confirm/exclude the presence of intramyocardial fibrosis; postcontrast (15 min) T1 mapping for ECV calculation.

Main CMR Findings Volumes of the left ventricle are at the upper limit of normal with moderate reduction in global systolic function (LVEF = 38%).

Normal sizes, volumes, and function of the right ventricle with normal ejection fraction (RVEF = 68%) (Movie 2.12).

No signal abnormalities suggesting the presence of edema and no uptake of contrast agent in LGE images (no fibrotic tissue within the myocardium).

The T1 mapping values are slightly elevated with interstitial volumes (ECV) at the upper limits, possibly related to the expansion of the interstitial space.

T1 mapping value (ShMOLLI) 1025 ± 28 ms (normal values 962 ± 25 ms) (Piechnik et al. JCMR 2013) (Piechnik et al. JCMR 2013).

Extracellular volume: 29% (normal values 25 ± 3%) (Fontana et al. JCMR 2012).

Conclusion The pathologic findings can be related to the previous chemo- and radiotherapy.

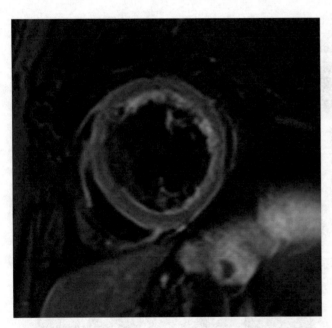

Fig. 2.16 T2-weighted image. Short-axis view of the heart. No signal abnormalities are detectable

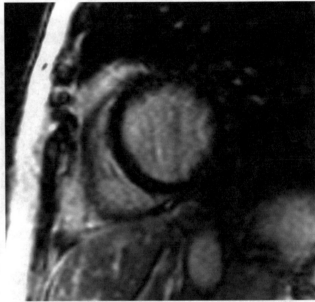

Fig. 2.17 Late gadolinium enhancement GRE-IR image. No areas of contrast agent uptake are detectable

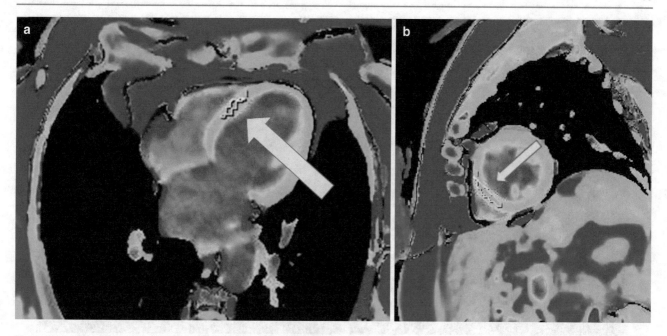

Fig. 2.18 Precontrast T1 mapping image. (**a**) Horizontal long axis and (**b**) midventricular short axis. Abnormally long T1 is detected at the level of the interventricular septum within the region of interest indicated by the arrow

2.4   Post-transcatheter Ablation Scar

Male, 15 y.o. Familiarity positive for sudden cardiac death. History of sustained ventricular tachycardia and transcatheter ablation. Currently evidence of extrasystolic activity.

CMR Flowchart   Stack of cine images in short-axis view to evaluate biventricular volumes and function. LGE GRE-IR images to detect the presence of pathologic uptake of c.a.

Main CMR Findings   Normal biventricular global and regional function (Movie 2.13). In LGE images evidence of focal fibrosis on the right-side interventricular septum where the previous transcatheter ablation was performed.

Conclusion   Postinterventional fibrosis.

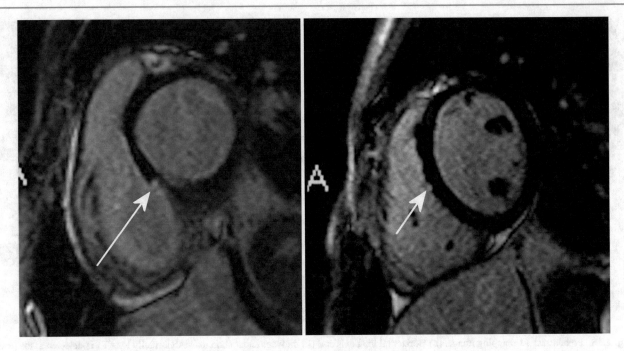

Fig. 2.19 Two LGE images in short axis. The arrows show the focal uptake of contrast agent in two small areas where presumably the transcatheter ablation was previously performed

2.5 Endomyocardial Fibrosis

2.5.1 Uncomplicated Endomyocardial Fibrosis

Medical History Male, 22 y.o. Originally from Central Africa. In the last months repeated feverish episodes. Increased eosinophilia. Heart failure. Long-lasting warfarin therapy.

CMR Flowchart Stack of cine images in short-axis view to evaluate biventricular volumes and function. T2w images to assess the presence of myocardial edema. LGE images.

Main CMR Findings Increased left-ventricle volume (EDV = 128 ml/m², ESV = 85 ml/m²) and reduction of global function (EF: 33%) (Movie 2.14). Local abnormal signal in T2w images, diffuse subendocardial LGE, and some intramyocardial spotty uptake. No sign of intraventricular thrombosis.

Conclusion Endomyocardial fibrosis.

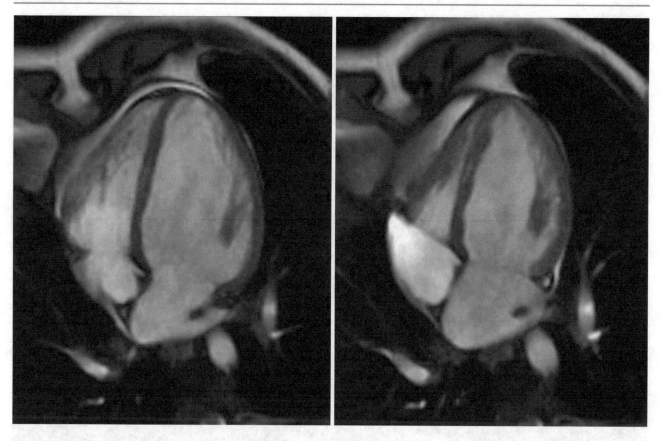

Fig. 2.20 SSFP cine images in horizontal long axis. Evidence of increased left-ventricle volumes and reduction of global ventricular function. Left panel: end-diastolic frame. Right panel: end-systolic frame

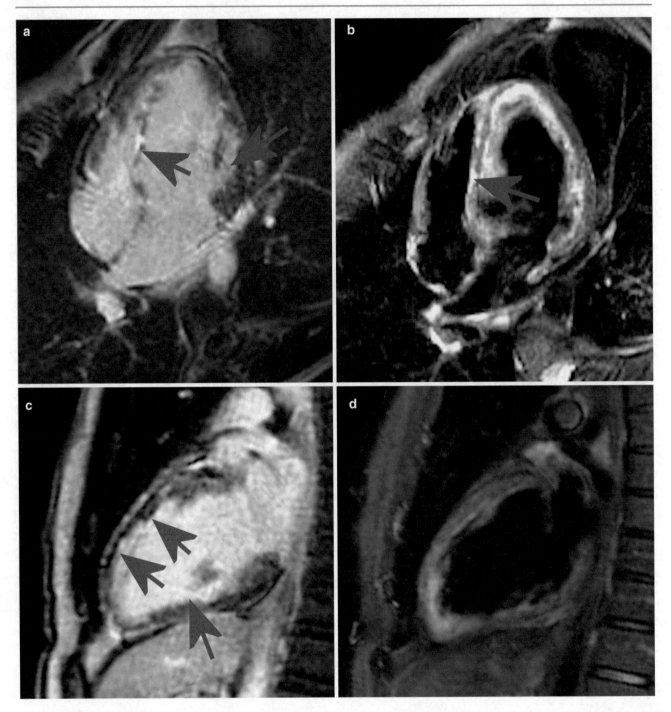

Fig. 2.21 LGE images (**a** and **c**) and T2w images (**b** and **d**). Upper panels in horizontal long-axis view. Lower panels (vertical long-axis view). In LGE images evidence of diffuse subendocardial uptake and some intramyocardial spotty deposits. In T2w images evidence of spotty intramyocardial edema

2.5.2   Endomyocardial Fibrosis with Intraventricular Thrombus

Medical History Female, 72 y.o. Chronic Obstructive Pulmonary Disease. Since 2 years increased counting of eosinophilic cells in blood samples. Asymptomatic. At Echocardiography suspect of intraventricular thrombus. At invasive angiography normal coronary arteries.

CMR Flowchart Stack of cine images in short-axis view to evaluate biventricular volumes and function. T2w images to assess the presence of myocardial edema. GRE-IR images (LGE technique). Acquisition after 3 and 10 min after the contrast agent administration.

Main CMR Findings Left-ventricle volume and global function normal. Increased thickness of the interventricular septum (13 mm). In long-axis view, the cine images show the presence of intraventricular thrombotic material at the level of the apex (Movie 2.15). No pathologic findings in T2w images. In GRE-IR images evidence of apical deposition of intraventricular material both in images acquired early (3 min, TI 355 ms) or late (10 min, TI 350 ms) after the contrast agent administration.

Conclusion Endomyocardial fibrosis with intraventricular thrombosis.

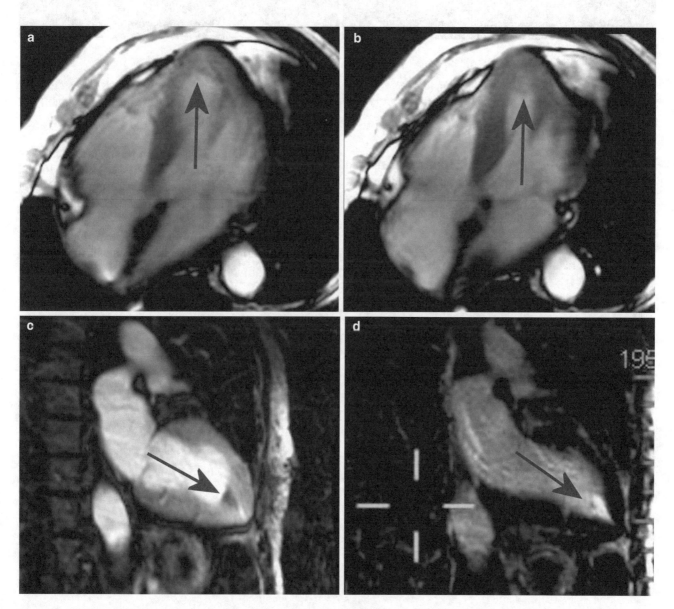

Fig. 2.22 (**a**) Long axis. SSFP cine sequence. Horizontal long axis diastolic frame (**b**) SSFP cine sequence. Horizontal long axis, systolic frame. (**c**) Vertical long axis. GRE-IR image acquired 3 min after contrast agent administration (0.15 mmol/kg). (**d**) Vertical long axis. GRE-IR image acquired 10 min after contrast agent administration. (**e**) Horizontal long axis. GRE-IR image acquired 3 min after contrast agent administration. (**f**) Horizontal long axis. Image acquired 10 min after contrast agent administration

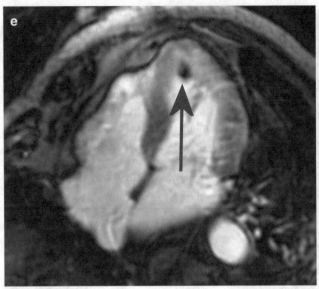
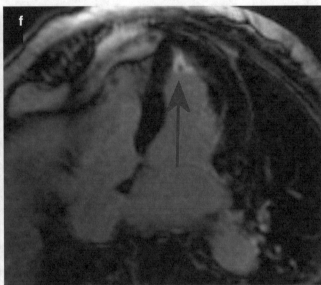

Fig. 2.22 (continued)

2.6   Cardiac Involvement in Systemic Lupus Erythematosus

Medical History   Female, 64 y.o. Since many years affected by lupus erythematosus, with moderate renal failure. At Echocardiography, evidence of light myocardial hypertrophy and initial impairment of global function.

CMR Flowchart   Stack of cine images in short-axis view to evaluate biventricular volumes and function. Stack of T2w images to assess the presence of myocardial edema. LGE images to detect myocardial fibrosis.

Main CMR Findings   Increased left ventricular volume and impairment of global function (EF 41%) (Movie 2.16 and Movie 2.17). No signal abnormalities in T2w images. Diffuse intramyocardial uptake of contrast agent in LGE images.

Conclusion   Cardiac involvement in systemic lupus erythematosus. Impairment of global function and diffuse myocardial fibrosis.

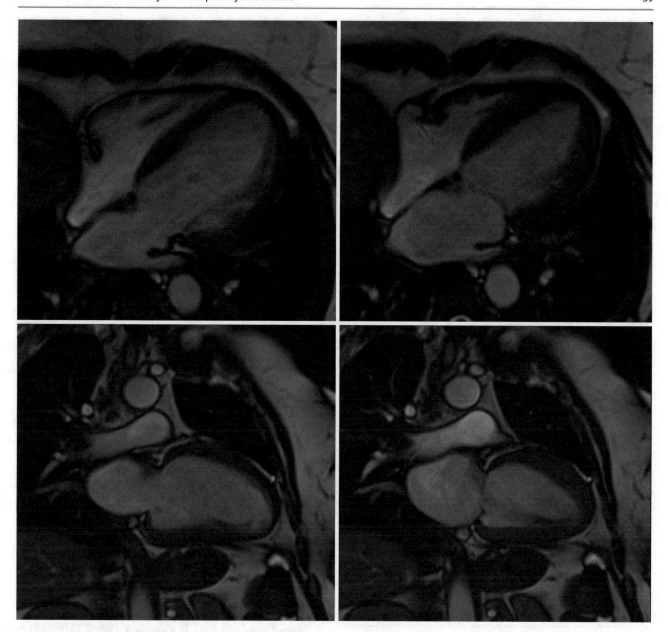

Fig. 2.23 SSFP cine images in horizontal (upper panels) and vertical long axis (lower panels). Left panels (end-diastolic frames); right panels (end-systolic frames). Evidence of increased volume and reduced function of left ventricle

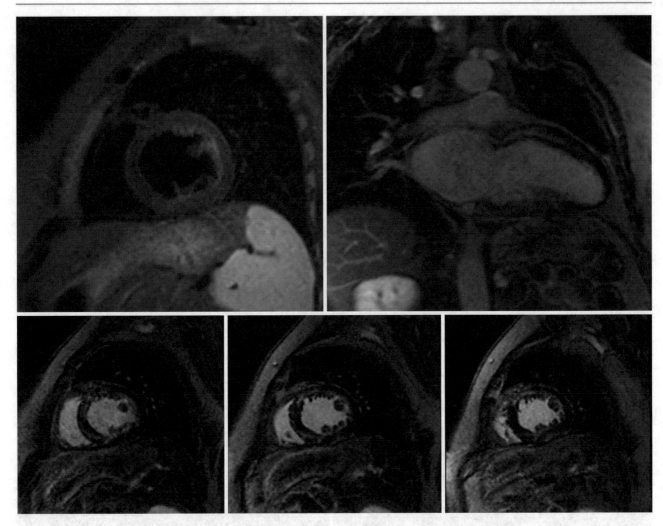

Fig. 2.24 Upper left panel: T2w image in short axis of the heart. No evidence of signal abnormalities. Upper right panel: LGE image in vertical long axis of the left ventricle. Intramyocardial contrast uptake either at the level of the interventricular septum and at the level of the inferior wall. Lower panels: LGE images. Three parallel short-axis views of the heart. Evidence of diffuse intramyocardial uptake of the contrast agent

Bibliography

1. Friedrich MG, Sechtem U, Schulz-Menger J, Holmvang G, Alakija P, Cooper LT, White JA, Abdel-Aty H, Gutberlet M, Prasad S, Aletras A, Laissy JP, Paterson I, Filipchuk NG, Kumar A, Pauschinger M, Liu P, International Consensus Group on Cardiovascular Magnetic Resonance in Myocarditis. Cardiovascular magnetic resonance in myocarditis: a JACC White Paper. J Am Coll Cardiol. 2009;53(17):1475–87.
2. Ferreira VM, Schulz-Menger J, Holmvang G, Kramer CM, Carbone I, Sechtem U, Kindermann I, Gutberlet M, Cooper LT, Liu P, Friedrich MG. Cardiovascular magnetic resonance in nonischemic myocardial inflammation: expert recommendations. J Am Coll Cardiol. 2018;72(24):3158–76.
3. Friedrich MG. Cardiovascular magnetic resonance for myocardial inflammation: Lake Louise versus mapping? Circ Cardiovasc Imaging. 2018;11(7):e008010.
4. Gannon MP, Schaub E, Grines CL, Saba SG. State of the art: evaluation and prognostication of myocarditis using cardiac MRI. J Magn Reson Imaging. 2019;49(7):e122–31.
5. Mukai-Yatagai N, Haruki N, Kinugasa Y, Ohta Y, Ishibashi-Ueda H, Akasaka T, Kato M, Ogawa T, Yamamoto K. Assessment of myocardial fibrosis using T1-mapping and extracellular volume measurement on cardiac magnetic resonance imaging for the diagnosis of radiation-induced cardiomyopathy. J Cardiol Cases. 2018;18(4):132–5.
6. Ferreira de Souza T, Quinaglia AC, Silva T, Osorio Costa F, Shah R, Neilan TG, Velloso L, Nadruz W, Brenelli F, Sposito AC, Matos-Souza JR, Cendes F, Coelho OR, Jerosch-Herold M, Coelho-Filho OR. Anthracycline therapy is associated with cardiomyocyte atrophy and preclinical manifestations of heart disease. JACC Cardiovasc Imaging. 2018;11(8):1045–55.
7. Kimball A, Patil S, Koczwara B, Raman KS, Perry R, Grover S, Selvanayagam J. Late characterisation of cardiac effects following anthracycline and trastuzumab treatment in breast cancer patients. Int J Cardiol. 2018;261:159–61.
8. Tao S, Guttman MA, Fink S, Elahi H, Patil KD, Ashikaga H, Kolandaivelu AD, Berger RD, Halushka MK, Schmidt EJ, Herzka DA, Halperin HR. Ablation lesion characterization in scarred substrate assessed using cardiac magnetic resonance. JACC Clin Electrophysiol. 2019;5(1):91–100.

9. Lombardi M, Plein S, Petersen S, Bucciarelli-Ducci C, Valsangiacomo-Buechel M, Basso C, Ferrari V. The EACVI textbook of cardiovascular magnetic resonance. Oxford: Oxford University Press; 2018.

10. Grimaldi A, Mocumbi AO, Freers J, Lachaud M, Mirabel M, Ferreira B, Narayanan K, Celermajer DS, Sidi D, Jouven X, Marijon E. Tropical endomyocardial fibrosis: natural history, challenges, and perspectives. Circulation. 2016;133(24):2503–15.

11. Mavrogeni S, Markousis-Mavrogenis G, Koutsogeorgopoulou L, Dimitroulas T, Bratis K, Kitas GD, Sfikakis P, Tektonidou M, Karabela G, Stavropoulos E, Katsifis G, Boki KA, Kitsiou A, Filaditaki V, Gialafos E, Plastiras S, Vartela V, Kolovou G. Cardiovascular magnetic resonance imaging pattern at the time of diagnosis of treatment naïve patients with connective tissue diseases. Int J Cardiol. 2017;236:151–6.

12. Burkard T, Trendelenburg M, Daikeler T, Hess C, Bremerich J, Haaf P, Buser P, Zellweger MJ. The heart in systemic lupus erythematosus—a comprehensive approach by cardiovascular magnetic resonance tomography. PLoS One. 2018;13(10):e0202105.

Ischemic Heart Disease

3.1 Acute Ischemic Heart Disease

3.1.1 Acute Myocardial Infarction

Clinical History 53-year-old male patient with the history of acute myocardial infarction treated by late PTCA and DES in LAD artery.

CMR Flowchart SSFP of cine images in vertical and horizontal long axes of the left ventricle. Stack of SSFP cine images in short axis to evaluate biventricular function. Same planes with T2w images to detect the eventual presence of myocardial edema and/or hemorrhage. Same planes with LGE (post-injection of gadolinium-based contrast agent; 0.2 mmol/kg) images to identify the extension and location of myocardial necrosis.

Main CMR Findings Normal sizes and volumes of the left ventricle. Wall thickness is mildly increased at the level of the interventricular septum. Impaired global LV function (LVEF = 35%) with large area of aki-dyskinesia in the territory of LAD (Movie 3.1, Movie 3.2 and Movie 3.3).

Normal sizes, volumes, and function of the right ventricle with normal ejection fraction (RVEF = 54%) with no regional function impairment.

Wide area of edema is noticed in T2 images with a central hypointense core interpreted as myocardial hemorrhage presumably due to the post-PTCA reperfusion.

In LGE images large area of the necrosis corresponding to the LAD territory. Within the necrotic area a large area of gross microvascular damage is noticed (no reflow). A small thrombotic mass at the level of left ventricle apex is not excludable.

Conclusion These findings describe an acute myocardial infarction in the LAD territory with large area of gross myocardial damage, and severe impairment of LV global left ventricular function.

Electronic Supplementary Material The online version of this chapter (https://doi.org/10.1007/978-3-030-41830-4_3) contains supplementary material, which is available to authorized users.

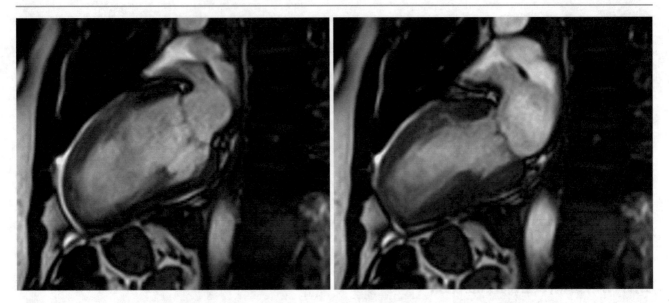

Fig. 3.1 SSFP cine images in vertical long-axis view of the left ventricle. A large aki-dyskinetic area corresponding to the territory of LAD is detectable. A severe impairment of global function is present. Left panel: end-diastolic frame. Right panel: end-systolic frame

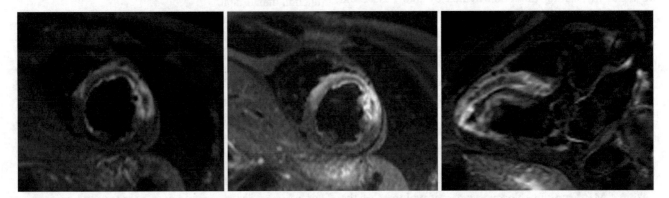

Fig. 3.2 T2w images. Left panel: proximal short axis of the left ventricle. Middle panel: midventricular short axis of the left ventricle. Right panel: vertical long axis of the left ventricle. In all the images a large area of myocardial hyperenhancement is detectable. Within the hyperenhanced area a large hypointense core is visible. This finding is interpretable as a large hemorrhagic area due to the post-PTCA reperfusion process

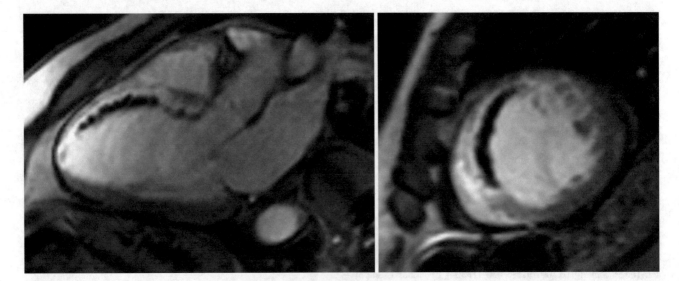

Fig. 3.3 LGE images obtained 10 min after the injection of gadolinium-based contrast agent (0.2 mmol/kg). A large necrotic area is detectable in the territory of LAD. Within the necrotic area (in white) large core of hypointense material is detectable interpreted as a gross myocardial damage (no reflow)

3.1.2 Acute Myocardial Infarction in Patient with a Previous Myocardial Infarction

Medical History Male, 58 y.o. Smoker, hypertension, hypercholesterolemia, hypothyroidism, familiarity for coronary artery disease.

Recent admission to the hospital because acute heart failure, at ECG LBB. At angiography significant stenosis of first marginal. Chronic total occlusion of right coronary artery with evidence of collateral circulation.

CMR Flowchart Cine images to evaluate ventricular function, T2w images to detect tissue characteristics of the recent myocardial infarction, LGE images to detect the presence of postischemic scar.

Main CMR Findings Large apical area of abnormal kinesis (dyskinesia) and reduced EF (41%) (Movie 3.4 and Movie 3.5). Evidence of myocardial edema in the territory of circumflex coronary artery (Acute Myocardial Infarction). Scar at the level of the inferior segments (Chronic Myocardial Infarction).

Conclusion Acute Myocardial Infarction in a patient with a previous Chronic Myocardial Infarction.

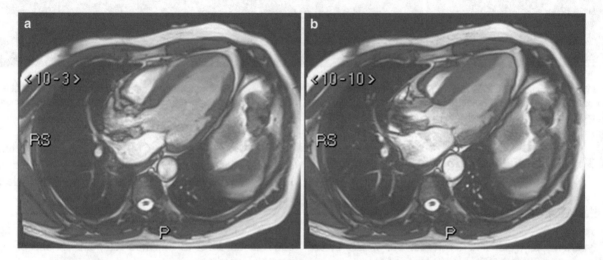

Fig. 3.4 Cine images. Diastolic (**a**) and systolic (**b**) frames in three-chamber view of left ventricle. Evidence of apical dyskinesia

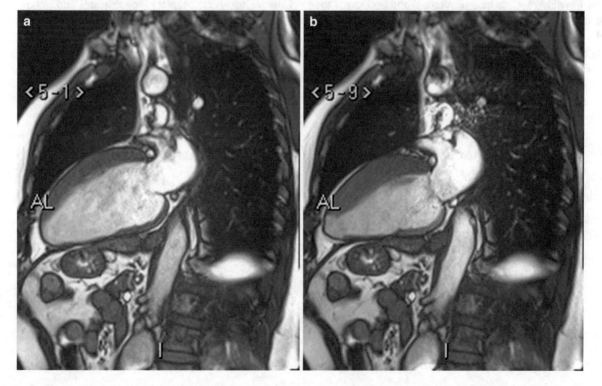

Fig. 3.5 Cine images. Diastolic (**a**) and systolic (**b**) frames in vertical long-axis view of left ventricle. Evidence of apical dyskinesia

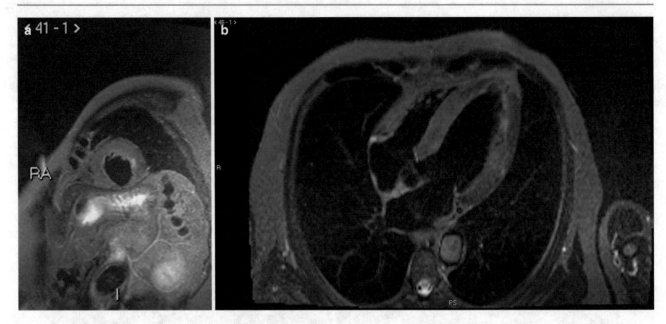

Fig. 3.6 T2w images (TR 2020 msec, TE 85 msec) in short axis (**a**) and horizontal long axis (**b**): evidence of a small subendocardial area with enhanced signal due to myocardial edema related to acute coro- nary syndrome in the territory of circumflex coronary artery that is in a different territory with respect to the chronic myocardia scar on the territory of posterior descending artery

3.1.3 Myocardial Infarction with Involvement of the Right Ventricle

Medical History Male, 59 y.o.

Hypertension, hypercholesterolemia. Six weeks before CMR, anterior STEMI. PTCA + STENT of LDA.

CMR Flowchart Cine images: vertical and horizontal long axis, thre chambers view, stack of short axis images to evaluate bi-ventricular regional and global function. T2w images to detect the presence of myocardial edema. LGE images to detect the presence and exension of myocardial scar.

Main CMR Findings At CMR: Akinesia of left ventricle septal segments in mid and apical segments. Akinesia of inferior and diaphragmatic segments of right-ventricle free wall. (Movie 3.6 and Movie 3.7)

LGE images show transmural uptake of contrast agent either at the level of impaired left-ventricle and of right-ventricle segments.

Conclusion Anteroseptal myocardial infarction with involvement of the right-ventricle free wall.

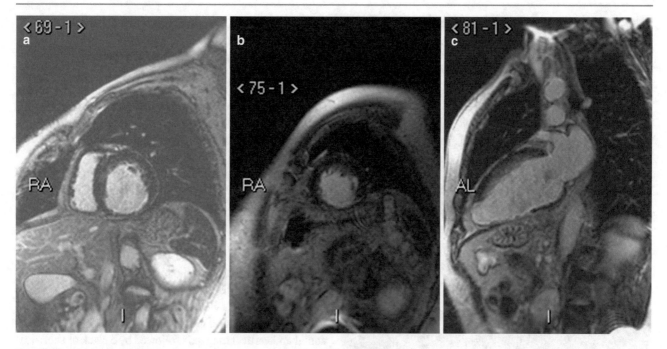

Fig. 3.7 LGE images. Short-axis view at proximal (**a**) and at midventricle level (**b**). Evidence of c.a. uptake at lateral segment (circumflex territory) indicative of altered c.a. kinetic. In **a**, in **b**, and in **c** evidence of inferior scar

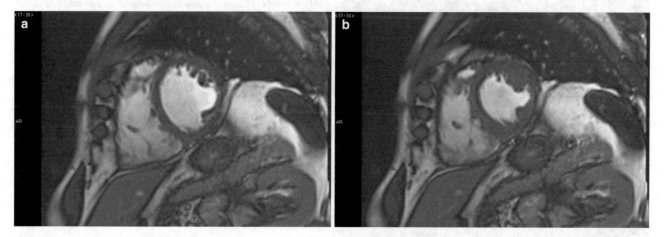

Fig. 3.8 Cine images in short axis of the heart. (**a**) Diastolic frame, (**b**) systolic frame. Evidence of large akinetic area involving the septal segments of left ventricle and the diaphragmatic segment of the right ventricle

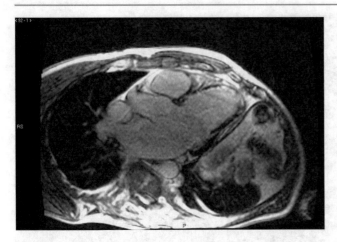

Fig. 3.9 Late postcontrast GRE-IR image (LGE). Three-chamber view. Large necrotic area at the level of the anterior segments

3.2   Chronic Coronary Artery Disease

3.2.1   Previous Myocardial Infarction

Clinical History Forty-three-years-old female. Ex-smoker with family history of coronary artery disease. Five years earlier acute coronary syndrome followed by coronary angiography which showed nonsignificant stenosis of the LAD. Treated with optimal medical therapy.

Last echocardiogram showed normal ejection fraction of the left ventricle (LVEF = 64%) and akinesia of the apex, and hypokinesia of the inferior apical wall. No significant valvular pathology.

At Holter ECG: minor ventricular arrhythmias.

CMR Flowchart SSFP cine images in horizontal and vertical long axis of the left ventricle followed by a stack of images in short-axis view of the left ventricle to evaluate volumes and regional and global function. LGE images in horizontal and vertical long axis followed by a stack of short-axis images to evaluate the presence, location, and extension of myocardial scar.

MR Report Normal sizes and volumes of the left ventricle. Akinesia of the anteroseptal and anterior wall in basal segments. Dyskinesia of apical segments (anterior, septum, inferior). Mild reduction of the left ventricular global function (LVEF = 49%) (Movie 3.8 and Movie 3.9).

Normal range of the sizes, volumes, and function of the right ventricle.

Presence of transmural scar in the territory of the LAD.

Conclusion Previous myocardial infarction on the territory of LAD. Mild reduction of global LV function.

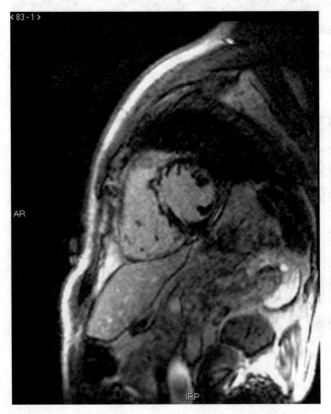

Fig. 3.10 Late postcontrast GRE-IR image (LGE). Short-axis view. Evidence of necrotic area at the level of the anteroseptal segment and the diaphragmatic segment of the right ventricle

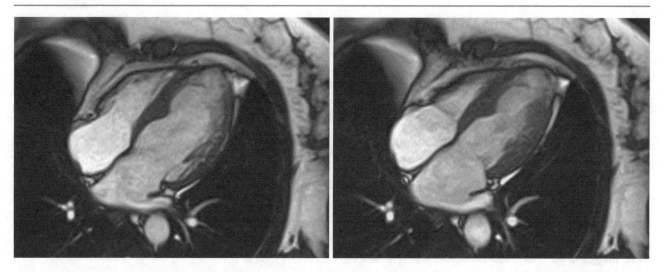

Fig. 3.11 SSFP cine images in horizontal long axis. Left panel: end-diastolic frame. Right panel: end-systolic frame. Evidence of impairment of function at the level of apical segments which appear thinned and aki-dyskinetic

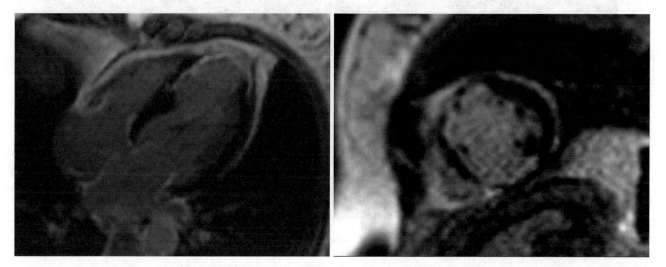

Fig. 3.12 LGE images in horizontal long axis (left panel) and short axis (right panel). Evidence of almost transmural uptake (50–100% of transmurality) at the level of the apical segments

3.2.2 Postischemic Cardiomyopathy

Clinical History Male, 88 y.o. Ex-smoker, with a history of arterial hypertension, and inferior posterolateral myocardial infarction treated by PTCA on proximal circumflex coronary artery.

In the follow-up the patient was admitted to ER because of severe dyspnea and heart failure. Echocardiogram showed dilation of the left ventricle with large akinesia at the level of the proximal and mid inferior and inferolateral segments. Severe impairment of global function of LV with an EF = 33%. Right ventricle dilated and globally hypokinetic.

CMR Flowchart Stack of cine images in short-axis view to evaluate biventricular volumes and function. Postcontrast LGE images in short-axis and horizontal and vertical long-axis views.

Main CMR Findings Dilated left ventricle, with severely depressed systolic function (LVEF = 26%) with global hypokinesia and akinesia of inferior and inferolateral walls (Movie 3.10).

Right-ventricle sizes and volumes are at the upper limits of normal with severely depressed systolic function (RVEF = 27%) with global hypokinesia (Movie 3.10).

In postcontrast LGE images a large scar is detectable in the territory of the circumflex coronary artery. The scar involves the inferior and inferolateral wall with 75–100% of transmurality and low likelihood of viable myocardium.

Conclusion Postischemic cardiomyopathy, large postischemic scar, and no viable myocardium.

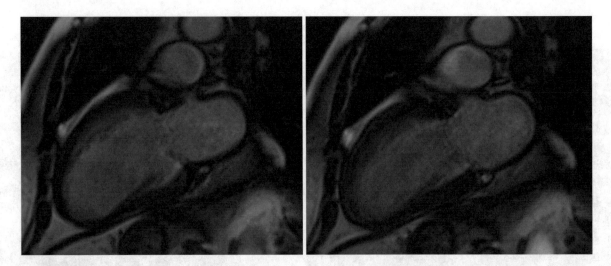

Fig. 3.13 SSFP cine images in vertical long-axis view. Left panel: end-diastolic frame; right panel: end-systolic frame

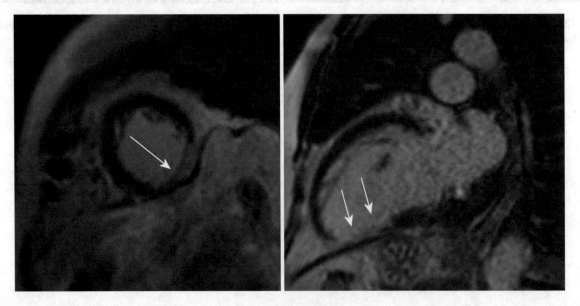

Fig. 3.14 Postcontrast LGE images. Left panel: short-axis view of left ventricle. Right panel: vertical long axis view of the left ventricle. The arrows show the scar tissue as evidenced by LGE

3.2.3 Complicated Myocardial Infarction

3.2.3.1 Postischemic Cardiomyopathy with Intraventricular Thrombus

Clinical History Male, 54 y.o. History of ischemic cardiomyopathy with chronic total occlusion of left anterior descending artery (LAD) and multiple stenosis of other coronary arteries.

Dyspnea during moderate effort.

An echocardiographic examination, performed 2 years before the CMR examination, showed a LVEF of 43%. Previous episode of atrial flutter.

CMR Flowchart Cine images in vertical and horizontal long axis of left ventricle. Stack of cine images in short-axis view to evaluate biventricular volumes and function. LGE images after injection of gadolinium-based c.a. (0.2 mmol/kg) with optimized TI to view the localization and extension of the necrotic area and long TI for a better view of the intraventricular thrombus.

Main CMR Findings Increased left ventricular volume (107 ml/m²). Moderate reduction of left ventricular function (EF 40%) and presence of large apical aneurism. Large apical thrombus (Movie 3.11).

Conclusion Postischemic cardiomyopathy with large necrotic area and apical aneurism and intraventricular thrombus.

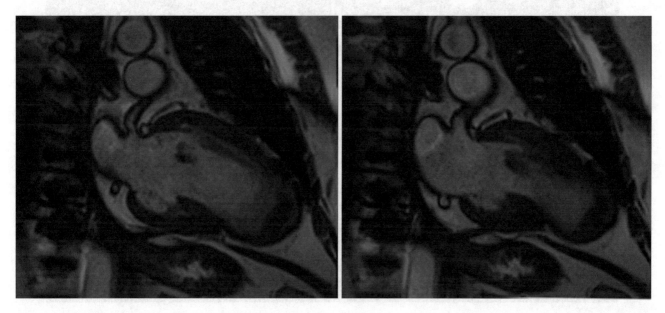

Fig. 3.15 Cine images of left ventricle vertical long axis. Evidence of a large apical aneurism with suspected intraventricular thrombus. Left panel: end-diastolic frame. Right panel: end-systolic frame

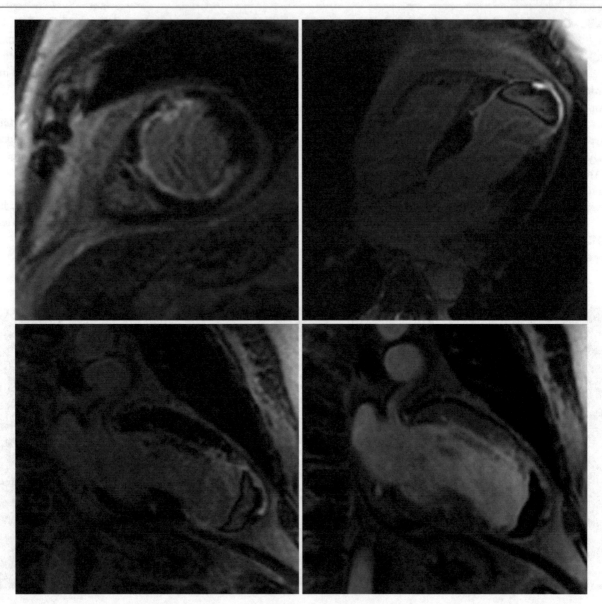

Fig. 3.16 LGE images with optimized TI for a better definition of the necrotic area. Left upper panel: midventricular short axis; right panel: horizontal long axis; left lower panel: vertical long axis. LGE image with prolonged TI (450 ms) (lower right panel) for a better nulling of the signal from the thrombotic mass

3.2.3.2 Cardiac Rupture

Medical History   Male, 81 y.o. First heart attack (AMI) at the age of 54 years. At further AMI, at the age of 71 years, treated by PTCA and STENT. Unstable angina 1 year after and a further PTCA and STENT. During routine cardiac assessment evidence at Echocardiography of a large para-cardiac mass.

CMR Flowchart   Stack of cine images in short-axis view to evaluate biventricular volumes and function and to assess the morphology and dimension of the para-cardiac mass. SSFP cine images in long-axis and oblique view to assess morphology, dimensions, and mechanical consequences of the para-cardiac mass. LGE images to assess the presence and extension of the previous AMIs and to characterize the para-cardiac mass.

Main CMR Findings   Normal left-ventricle volume. Impaired global function (EF: 40%) in the presence of akinesia at the level of the midventricle inferior wall and hypokinesia at the level of the midventricle lateral segments. Evidence of a transmural myocardial infarction at the level of the midventricle inferior wall. The myocardial thickness at this level appears extremely reduced. Presence of a large para-cardiac mass at the level of the inferior and posterior segments (Movie 3.12 and Movie 3.13). The content of the mass appears to be quite inhomogeneous both in SSFP cine images and in LGE images.

Conclusion   Chronic rupture of the heart. Confirmed by the Surgeon.

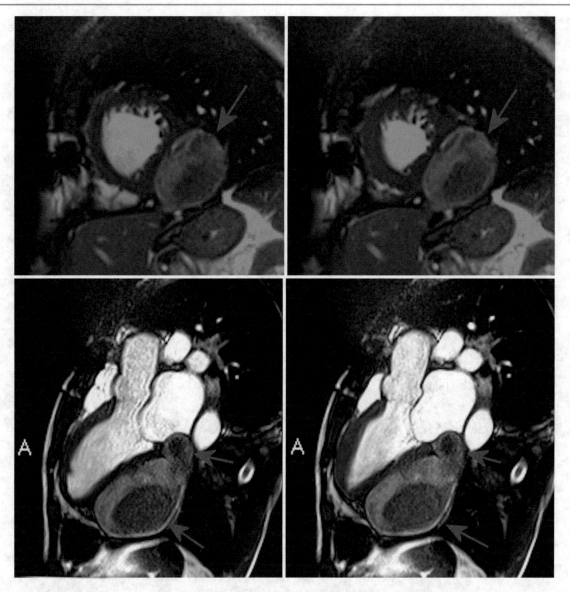

Fig. 3.17 Upper panels: SSFP images in short-axis view of the heart. Evidence of a dis-homogeneous round-shaped mass (arrows) at the level of the inferior segments. Lower panels: three-chamber view of the left ventricle. The mass shows a bilobar shape (arrows). Left panels in end diastole and right panels in end systole

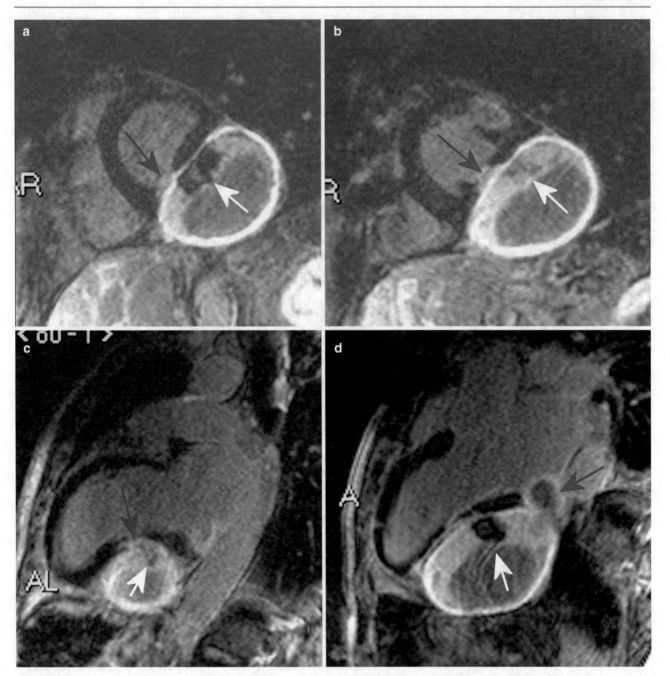

Fig. 3.18 LGE image. (**a** and **b**) Two contiguous slices of the heart in short-axis view. The red arrows show the myocardial infarction at the level of the inferior wall. The white arrows show thrombotic material. (**c**) Vertical long-axis view. The red arrow shows the thinned necrotic tissue due to the previous myocardial infarction. In (**d**): three-chamber view with evidence of a second, round-shaped, section of the mass (red arrow). The white arrow shows the thrombotic material inside the paracardiac mass

3.2.3.3 Left-Ventricle Pseudo-Aneurism

Medical History Male, 76 y.o. One year earlier AMI with evidence of total occlusion of Cx.

CMR Flowchart Stack of cine images in short-axis view to evaluate biventricular volumes and function. Cine images in oblique view to obtain diagnostic images at the level of the lateral wall. Postcontrast LGE images.

Main CMR Findings Increased left-ventricle volume with reduced global function (EF 32%). Presence of a large pseudo-aneurismatic structure at the level of the midventricle lateral wall (Movie 3.14, Movie 3.15 and Movie 3.16).

Conclusion Left-ventricle postischemic pseudo-aneurism and reduced global function.

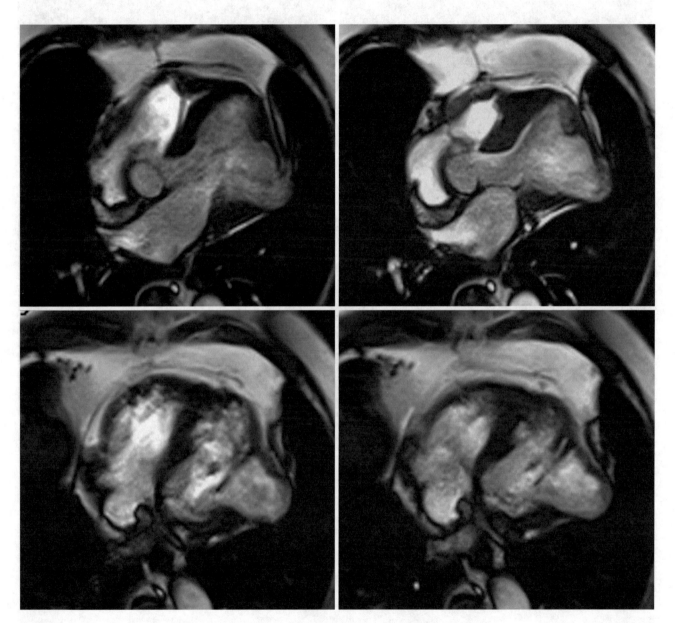

Fig. 3.19 SSFP cine images in three-chamber view (upper panels and in horizontal long-axis (mid panels) and in short-axis view at midventricle (lower panels). Vertical long axis (middle panels) and horizontal long axis (lower panels). Left panels in end-diastolic phase. Right panels in end-systolic phase. Evidence of a large pseudo-aneurismatic structure communicating with the left ventricle cavity. The wall of the pseudo-aneurism is either very thinned or absent

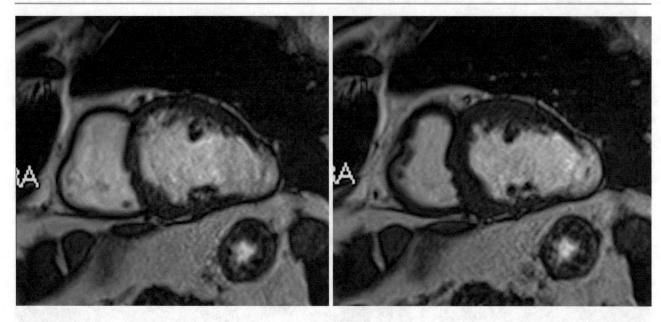

Fig. 3.19 (continued)

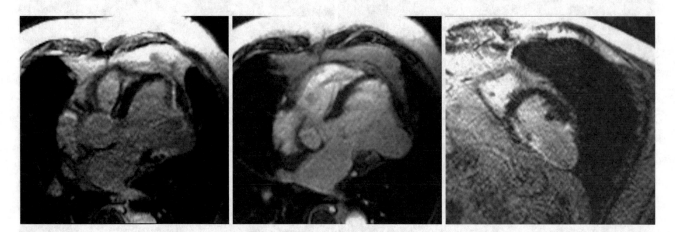

Fig. 3.20 Postcontrast LGE images. Evidence of uptake of the contrast agent at the level of the proximal inferolateral wall. The thin wall surrounding the pseudo-aneurism shows a diffuse albeit variable uptake of the contrast agent. Left panel: three-chamber view, mid panel: horizontal long-axis view, right panel: short-axis view

3.3   Stress CMR

3.3.1   Myocardial Inducible Ischemia in Stable CAD

Medical History Male, 72 y.o. Previous PCA + stent on CDx. Normal global function at Echocardiography. Typical chest pain on effort.

CMR Flowchart Stack of cine images in short-axis view to evaluate biventricular volumes, function, and wall thickness. Perfusion images: three slices in short axis view of the left ventricle acquired every beat during the first pass of a bolus of Gd-based contrast agent (0.075 mmol/kg). First pass evaluated during adenosine infusion (140 μg/min × 6 min) and in baseline conditions. LGE images in short-axis view.

Main CMR Findings Left-ventricle volume and global function normal (Movie 3.17).

During adenosine infusion, typical chest pain. Transmural area of hypoperfusion at inferolateral and inferior walls in midventricle slice and lateral wall in the distal slice (Movie 3.18).

Conclusion Inducible ischemia in the territory of circumflex-marginal branch confirmed by angiography.

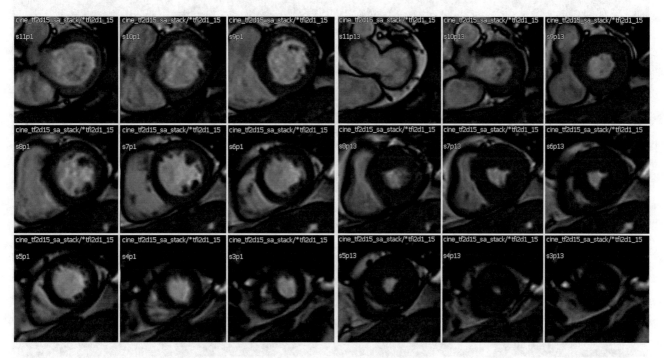

Fig. 3.21 Stack of SSFP cine images in short axis covering the whole heart. Normal global function and no regional wall motion abnormalities (the three colums on the left in end diastole, the three columns on the right in end systole).

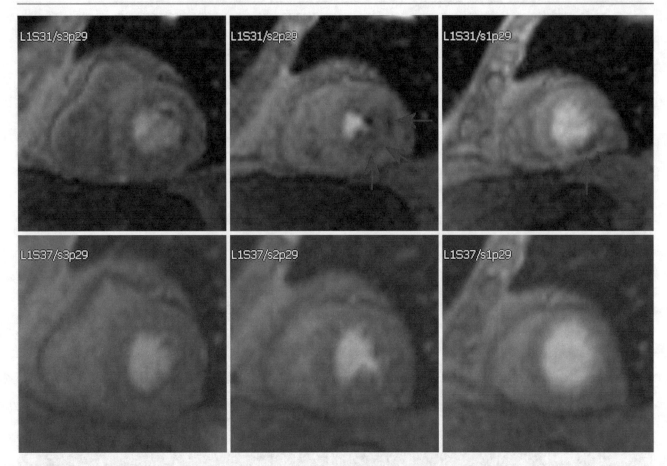

Fig. 3.22 Perfusion images (IR-GRE) obtained during the first pass through the heart of a bolus of contrast agent i.v. injected. Evidence of a transmural hypoperfused area at the level of the inferolateral and inferior wall in the midventricle and in the distal slice

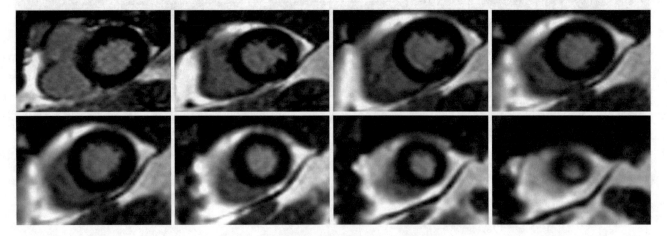

Fig. 3.23 Stack of LGE images in short-axis view of the heart. No evidence of myocardial uptake of c.a.

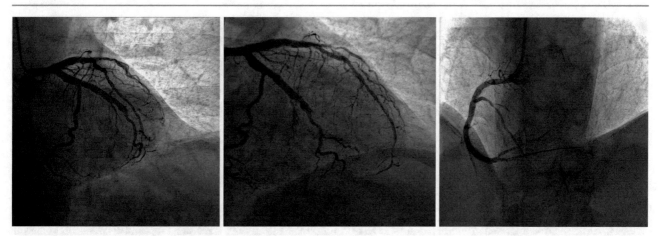

Fig. 3.24 Coronary angiography. Radial approach. Evidence of total chronic occlusion of the posterolateral branch. Minor stenosis on distal LAD. Significant stenosis at the level of interventricular posterior branch

3.3.2 Stress Test in Patient with Previous CABG

Clinical History 76-year-old male patient with the history of diabetes mellitus and arterial hypertension. In 1988 CABG. In 1991 recurrence of angina pectoris. In 2002 redo CABG. In 2015 coronary CT showed graft (LIMA-LAD and Ao-D1-RCA) patency.

In 2012 scintigraphy showed inducible ischemia at the level of anteroseptal wall. The following coronary angiography showed patency of LIMA-LAD arterial graft and Saphenous Vein Graft/SVG) on RCA, while mild disease of Ao-D1 graft. Medical therapy was then optimized. Patient stable and seldom occurrence of angina.

CMR Flowchart Stack of cine images in short-axis view to evaluate biventricular volumes and function. Perfusion images (GRE-IR) acquired during first pass of a bolus of c.a. intravenously injected (0.075 mmol/kg). Postcontrast LGE images.

Main CMR Findings Normal biventricular regional and global function. Hypertrophy of the interventricular septum. Left ventricular EF 70%. During adenosine (140 µg/kg/min*6 min) inducible ischemia at the level of the anterior anteroseptal wall (proximal, mid, and apical segments) (Movie 3.19). No evidence of scar at late gadolinium enhancement images.

Conclusion Stress CMR with adenosine positive for the presence of inducible ischemia in anteroseptal segments.

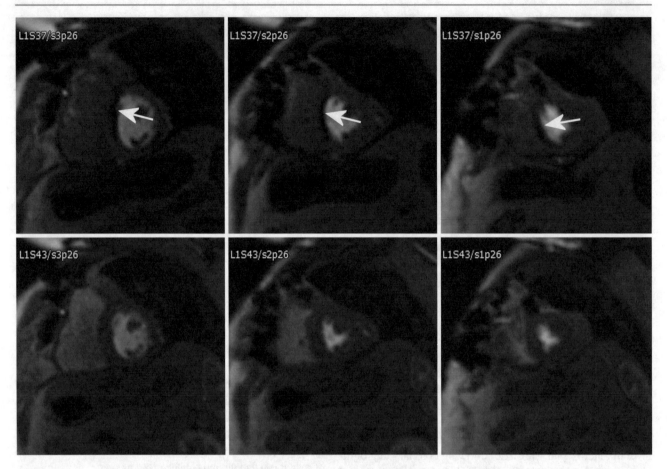

Fig. 3.25 Perfusion images obtained under adenosine infusion (upper panels) (140 µg/kg/min/6 min) and at baseline (lower panels) during the first pass of a bolus of contrast agent (0.075 mmol (kg)). The arrows show the presence of inducible ischemia at the level of the anteroseptal inferoseptal segments

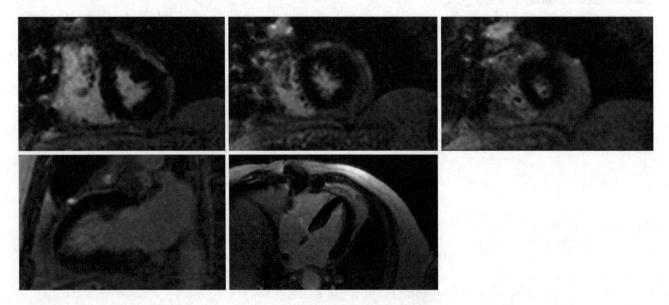

Fig. 3.26 Postcontrast LGE images obtained 10 min after the injection of c.a. (0.15 mmol/kg). No areas of uptake are detectable

3.3.3 Stress Cardiac Magnetic Resonance in Previous Myocardial Infarction

Medical History 83 y.o. Female. Risk factors: Familiarity, hypertension, hypercholesterolemia. Previous inferior myocardial infarction. Treadmill effort test negative for inducible ischemia.

CMR Flowchart Stack of cine images in short-axis view to evaluate biventricular volumes and function. Perfusion images: three slices in short axis of the left ventricle acquired during the first pass of a bolus of Gd-based contrast agent (0.075 mmol/kg). First pass evaluated during adenosine infusion (140 µg/min × 6 min) and in baseline conditions. LGE images in short-axis view.

Main CMR Findings Area of impaired regional function at the level of inferior and inferolateral segments with normal global function (Movie 3.20 and Movie 3.21). During pharmacological stress test an area of hypoperfusion corresponding to inferoseptal, inferior, and inferolateral segments is detectable (Movie 3.22). In LGE images an area of myocardial necrosis at the level of inferoseptal and inferior level is detectable. Significant discrepancy between the extension of the necrotic area and the extension of the hypoperfused area.

Conclusion Impairment of regional function but preserved global function of left ventricle. Previous myocardial infarction involving inferior and inferoseptal segments. Stress test positive for inducible ischemia in the same segments but with a larger extension with respect to the necrotic area.

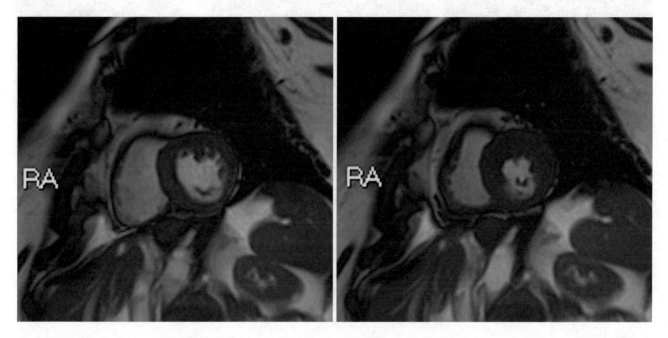

Fig. 3.27 Cine images. Left panel end-diastolic frame, right panel end-systolic frame. Evidence of akinesia at the level of inferior inferolateral segments

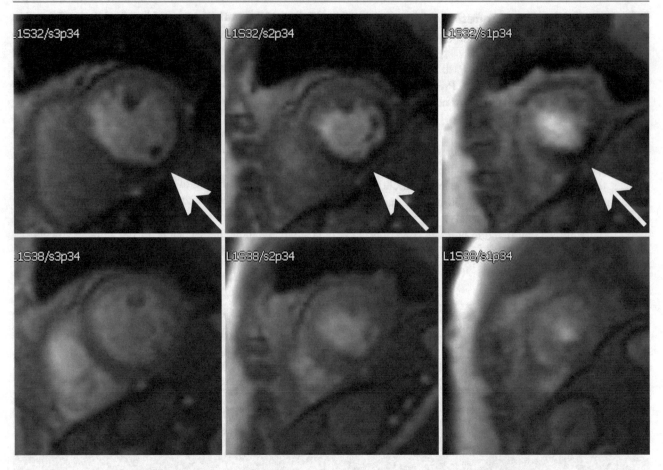

Fig. 3.28 Perfusion images. Upper panels during pharmacological stress (adenosine 140 microgamma/kg/min∗6 min). Three parallel slices (proximal, mid ventricle and apical view). The arrows show the transmural perfusion defects at the level of inferior, inferoseptal, and inferolateral walls. Lower panels: perfusion images acquired in baseline conditions showing no underperfused segments

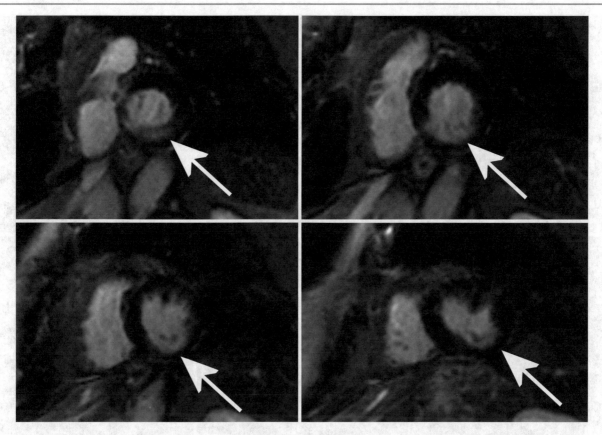

Fig. 3.29 LGE images in short axis view of the left ventricle. Four parallel slices. Upper left panel: proximal slice. Right upper panel: mid-ventricular view. Lower left panel: midventricular view. Lower right panel: short axis at the level of the apical segments. The arrows show the late gadolinium enhancement involving the inferior, inferoseptal, and inferolateral segments. However the extension of LGE is much smaller than the perfusion defect

3.3.4   Stress Cardiac Magnetic Resonance in Previous Myocardial Infarction and Coronary Artery Chronic Total Occlusion (CTO)

Clinical History 49-year-old male patient with a history of arterial hypertension and dyslipidemia. In 2012 inguinal hernioplasty. In presurgical check an abnormal ECG was recorded (Q wave in anterior leads). At echocardiogram LVEF of 50%, and hypokinesia of anterior apical wall. Effort stress test negative. Myocardial SPECT reported apical necrosis and perinecrotic inducible ischemia. Coronary angiography showed three-vessel disease with chronic total occlusion of LAD and LCX distal, critical stenosis of the first diagonal branch, RCA and LCX proximal.

CMR Flowchart SSFP stack of cine images in short axis view to evaluate global and regional function. GRE-IR perfusion images (three slices) during infusion of adenosine (140 μg/kg∗6 min) and first pass of a bolus of 0.075 mmol/kg of i.v.-administered Gd-based contrast agent. The same perfusion sequence with contrast agent bolus was also repeated 10 min after the stress. LGE images.

Main CMR Findings Normal volumes of the left ventricle, with systolic function at the lower normal limits (LVEF = 54%). Presence of wall motion abnormalities at the inferior and inferolateral segments.

Right-ventricle sizes, volumes, and systolic function are within the normal range.

Presence of transmural necrosis at inferior and inferolateral segments.

During the infusion of adenosine evidence of perfusion defect corresponding to the zone of necrosis and the presence of ischemia at the proximal-mid inferolateral wall segments. An adjunctive small area of ischemia is detectable at the level of the anteroseptal proximal wall (Movie 3.23).

Stress CMR was reported as positive for induceable ischemia in the proximal and mid inferolateral segment and in anteroseptal proximal segment. Presence of viable myocardium at the level of lateral segments.

Conclusion The positive stress test with the presence of viable myocardium suggested to proceed with transcatheter reopening of CTOs.

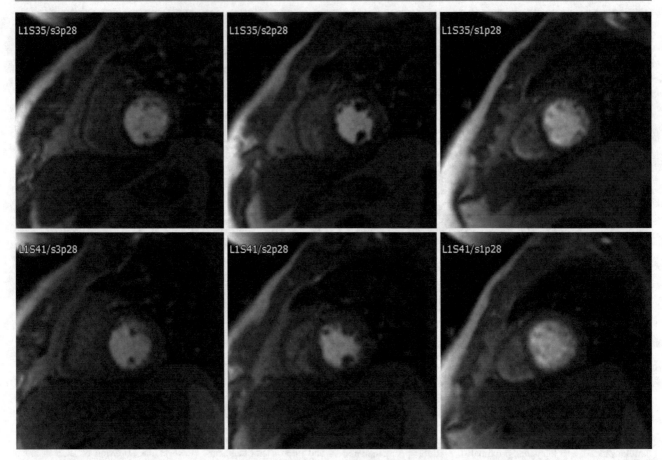

Fig. 3.30 Still frame from a perfusion sequence. First-pass technique. Upper panel: images obtained during adenosine stress. Evidence of a large area of hypoperfusion involving the inferior, inferoseptal, and inferolateral segments. Lower panel: images obtained in baseline condition with no evidence of hypoperfused areas

Fig. 3.31 Time-intensity curves obtained by the middle image in short-axis view (upper panel of Fig. 3.30). Two of the six segments (S1 and S2 corresponding to the inferior and inferolateral segments) show a slower enhancement (reduced slope of the curve during the wash-in phase) during the first pass of the contrast media through the myocardium. The wash-in slope can be utilized for a semiquantitative evaluation of perfusion (2)

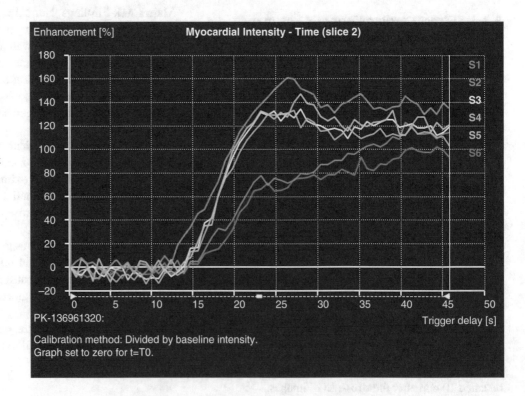

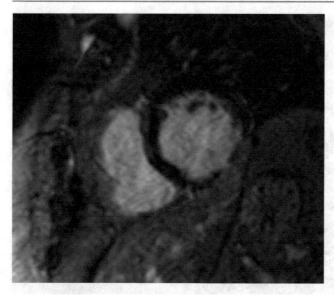

Fig. 3.32 LGE GR-IR images showing necrotic area involving the inferior and inferolateral segments. The necrosis is only partially transmural

3.3.5 Dobutamine Stress: Ischemia Assessment (Regional Function and Regional Perfusion)

Clinical History Male, 71 y.o. Patient with multiple cardiovascular risk factors: smoker, diabetes mellitus, hypertension, dyslipidemia.

At the age of 53 y.o.: anterior STEMI and PTCA on LAD. At the age of 61 y.o: PTCA on LAD because of intrastent stenosis. At the age of 65 y.o.: inferior STEMI treated by PTCA on RCA.

One year earlier: angina pectoris treated by PTCA on LCX and marginal branch, residual chronic total occlusion of RCA.

Residual angina by effort.

At Echocardiography left ventricle's sizes are at normal range with hypokinesia of the inferior wall mid-apical segment in the presence of thinning of wall. Preserved ejection fraction, no valvular dysfunction.

CMR Flowchart Stack of cine images in a short-axis view for evaluation of regional and global function at baseline. The same cine images are repeated during each stage of the administration of dobutamine (5, 10, 20, 30 gamma/kg b.w.). Evaluation of perfusion (first-pass technique with the i.v. injection of Gd-based contrast agent: 0.075 mmol/kg for each injection) at baseline and at maximum heart rate (135 b/min). LGE images at the end of the study.

Main CMR Findings Normal sizes, volumes, and function of the left ventricle; the wall thickness at the level of the interventricular septum is mildly increased. Normal ejection fraction (LVEF = 63%) with no clear regional wall motion abnormalities (Movie 3.24 and Movie 3.25).

Normal sizes, volumes, and function of the right ventricle with normal ejection fraction (RVEF = 68%) with no contractility impairment.

During the dobutamine infusion progressive improvement of global function is detectable (Fig. 3.33). No regional wall motion abnormalities at higher dosage with hyperkinetic response of the whole left ventricle (Movie 3.26).

No perfusion abnormalities were detected in baseline conditions. At the peak of the dobutamine infusion, perfusion defect in anterior and anterolateral wall mid distal segments was observed which partially corresponds to the zone of previous myocardial infarction (necrotic area). A second ischemic territory was also detected at the level of the anterolateral segments (Movie 3.27).

In LGE images presence of necrotic tissue substantially nontransmural and with limited extension in the territory of the LAD and at the level of the inferior wall.

Findings referable to the presence of ischemia in the territory of LAD. A very limited extension of viable tissue in the territory of RCA.

Conclusion Good biventricular function. Two previous myocardial infarction either in the territory of LAD and in the territory of RCA without clear evidence of regional impairment of function. Inducible ischemia in the territory of LAD and RCA.

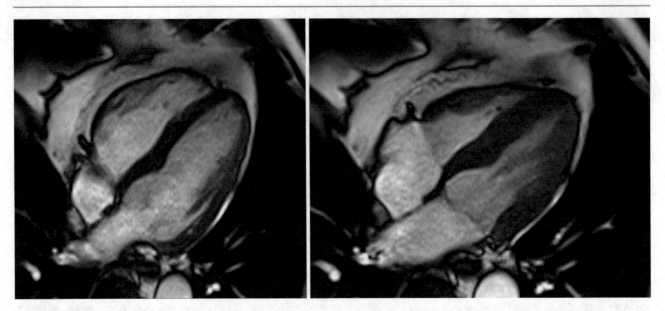

Fig. 3.33 SSFP cine images in horizontal long axis of the heart. Left panel: end-diastolic frame. Right panel: end-systolic frame

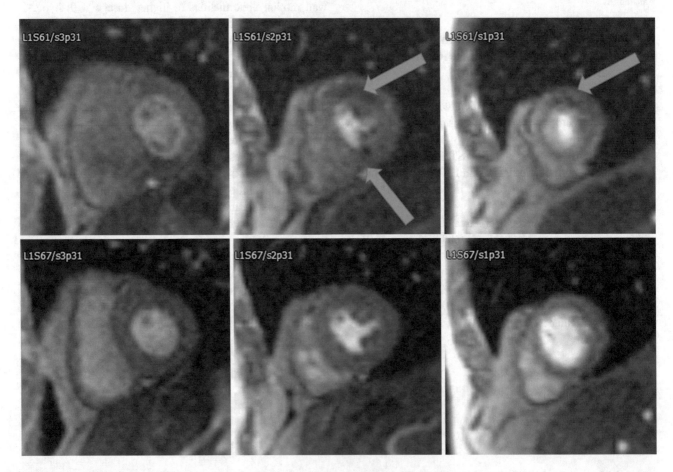

Fig. 3.34 Perfusion images (still frame at the peak of first pass of the contrast agent). The three upper images obtained at the top of dobutamine infusion. The three lower images obtained in baseline conditions. The arrows show the areas of induced hypoperfusion

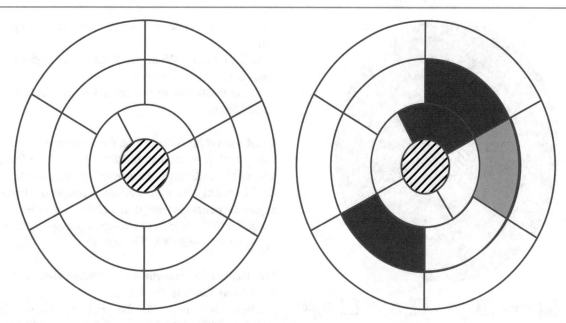

Fig. 3.35 Bull's eyes synthetizing the regional distribution of perfusion within each of the 17 segments of the left ventricle: completely normal at baseline and two different areas of hypoperfusion at the peak of the pharmacological stress (color code: white normal perfusion; light gray: nontransmural hypoperfusion (<50% of transmurality); dark gray: transmural hypoperfusion (>50% of transmurality) (Left panel at baseline, right panel at peak stress)

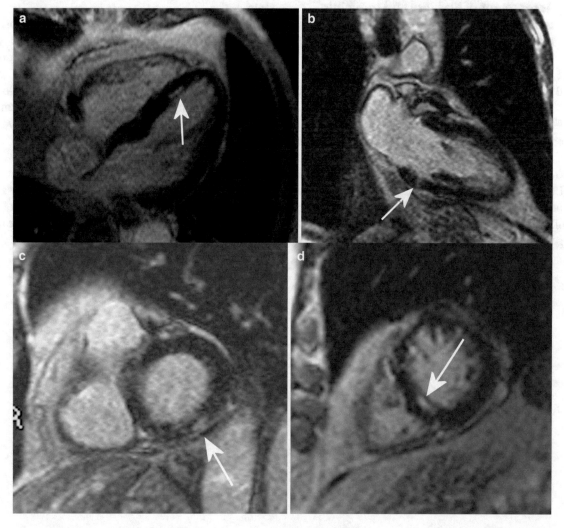

Fig. 3.36 LGE images left upper panel (**a**): horizontal long axis; right upper panel (**b**): vertical long axis; lower panels (**c** and **d**): two parallel short axes obtained at proximal and midventricular level. Arrows show areas of uptake of c.a. due to the previous episodes of myocardial infarction

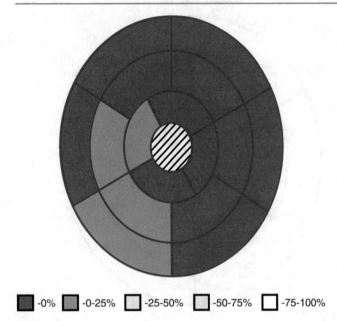

■ -0%   ■ -0-25%   ■ -25-50%   ■ -50-75%   □ -75-100%

Fig. 3.37 Bull's eye of the contrast agent uptake in LGE images. The color code indicates the transmurality of the uptake

3.3.6 Assessment of Viability and Inducible Ischemia in Previous Acute Myocardial Infarction

Clinical History 67-year-old male with the history of repeated revascularization procedures because of unstable angina.

In 1995 triple CABG (LIMA-AVI, SVG to AO-posterior interventricular artery (PIV) and AO-obtuse marginal branch).

In 2016 angiographic evidence of occlusion of the left main (LM), proximal stenosis of left and right coronary artery, occlusion of the graft of the obtuse marginal branch with collaterals for the left circumflex (LCX), occlusion of the graft for the posterior interventricular artery (IVP)

followed by percutaneous coronary reopening of LM and PIV.

In September 2018 angina followed by angioplasty (two drug-eluted stents) for LAD.

Stress CMR was recommended for the identification of the ischemia.

CMR Flowchart Stack of cine images to evaluate regional and global biventricular function. Same cine images are repeated at each stage of dobutamine administration (5, 10, 20, 30 gmma/kg/5 min. Perfusion image (first-pass technique) is performed at peak dobutamine effect. GRE-IR images during injection of Gd-based contrast agent at a dosage of 0.075 mmol/kg in 3 s. LGE images.

MR Report Conclusion Left-ventricle sizes and volumes at the lower limits of the normal.

Slight reduction of the left ventricular function (LVEF = 54%). Hypokinesia of the proximal anteroseptal segment and distal segment of the lateral wall. Akinesia of the basal-mid segments of the inferolateral wall (Movie 3.28).

Normal range of sizes, volumes, and function of the right ventricle.

Mild aortic and tricuspid regurgitation and stenosis.

Stress CMR: low-dosage dobutamine stress: (5 and 10 mg/kg/3–5 min) no improvement of preexisting regional abnormalities; at high dosage (20, 30, and 40 gamma/kg/3–5 min) (Movie 3.29) no evidence of wall motion worsening of preexisting or new onset of regional abnormalities.

In perfusion study there is clear evidence of hypoperfusion in the inferolateral and anteroseptal segments in correspondence of necrotic tissue (Movie 3.30).

Conclusion Absence of viable myocardium in the anterior, anteroseptal, and lateral wall with no evidence of stress-inducible ischemia in the territory not involved in the necrotic scar.

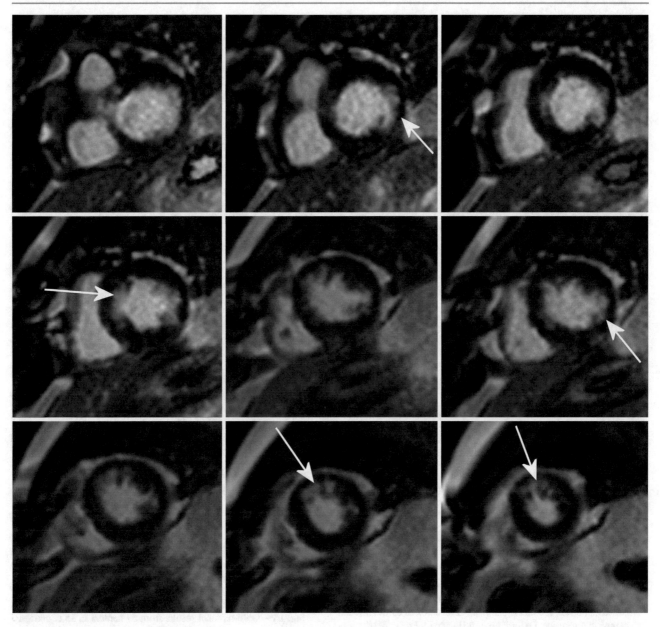

Fig. 3.38 GRE-IR LGE images in short axis of the left ventricles. Evidence of necrotic area in different coronary territories (arrows) with a variable between 25 and 75% of transmurality

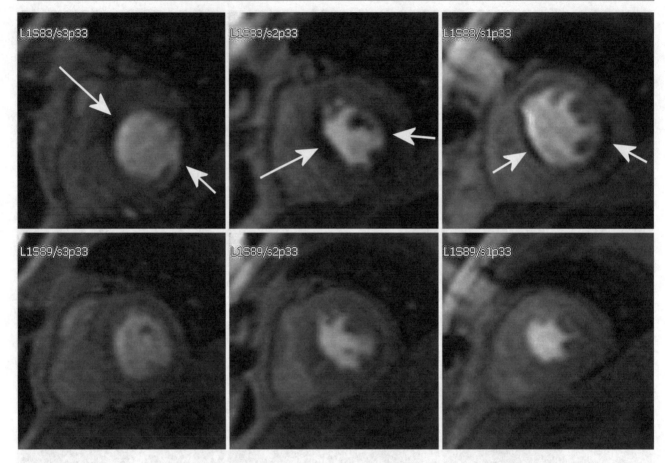

Fig. 3.39 Perfusion study (first-pass technique). Evidence of under-perfused areas in the same territories affected by ischemic scar. Upper panels: perfusion study during pharmacological stress (dobutamine 40 gamma/kg/5 min). Arrows show hypoperfused areas. Lower panels: perfusion study at baseline conditions

Bibliography

1. Gerber BL, et al. Chronic ischemic heart disease. In: Lombardi M, Plein S, Petersen S, Bucciarelli-Ducci C, Valsangiacoo Buechel M, Basso C, Ferrari V, editors. The EACVI textbook of cardiovascular magnetic resonance. Oxford: Oxford University Press; 2018.

2. Smulders MW, Bekkers SC, Kim HW, Van Assche LM, Parker MA, Kim RJ. Performance of CMR methods for differentiating acute from chronic MI. JACC Cardiovasc Imaging. 2015;8(6):669–79. https://doi.org/10.1016/j.jcmg.2014.12.030.

3. Masci PG, Marinelli M, Piacenti M, Lorenzoni V, Positano V, Lombardi M, L'Abbate A, Neglia D. Right ventricular ischemic injury in patients with acute ST-segment elevation myocardial infarction: characterization with cardiovascular magnetic resonance. Circ Cardiovasc Imaging. 2010;3(4):482–90.

4. Lombardi M, Plein S, Petersen S, Bucciarelli-Ducci C, Valsangiacomo-Buechel M, Basso C, Ferrari V. The EACVI Textbook of Cardiovascular Magnetic Resonance. Oxford; Oxford University Press; 2018.

5. Thomson LE, Kim RJ, Judd RM. Magnetic resonance imaging for the assessment of myocardial viability. J Magn Reson Imaging. 2004;19(6):771–88.

6. Waterhouse DF, Murphy TM, McCarthy J, O'Neill J, O'Hanlon R. LV apical rupture complicating acute myocardial infarction: the role of CMR. Heart Lung and Circ. 2015;24(7):e93–6.

7. Bruder O, Wagner A, Lombardi M, Schwitter J, van Rossum A, Pilz G, et al. European Cardiovascular Magnetic Resonance (EuroCMR) registry—multi-national results from 57 centers in 15 countries. J Cardiovasc Magn Reson. 2013;15:9.

8. Coelho-Filho OR, Seabra LF, Mongeon FP, Abdullah SM, Francis SA, Blankstein R, et al. Stress myocardial perfusion imaging by CMR provides strong prognostic value to cardiac events regardless of patient's sex. JACC Cardiovasc Imaging. 2011;4:850–61.

9. Al-Saadi N, Nagel E, Gross M, Bornstedt A, Schnackenburg B, Klein C, Klimek W, Oswald H, Fleck E. Noninvasive detection of myocardial ischemia from perfusion reserve based on cardiovascular magnetic resonance. Circulation. 2000;101(12):1379–83.

10. Pica S, Di Giovine G, Bollati M, Testa L, Bedogni F, Camporeale A, Pontone G, Andreini D, Monti L, Gasparini G, Grancini L, Secco GG, Maestroni A, Ambrogi F, Milani V, Lombardi M. Cardiac magnetic resonance for ischaemia and viability detection. Guiding patient selection to revascularization in coronary chronic total occlusions: The CARISMA_CTO study design. Int J Cardiol. 2018;272:356–62. https://doi.org/10.1016/j.ijcard.2018.08.061.

11. Löffler AI, Kramer CM. Myocardial viability testing to guide coronary revascularization. Interv Cardiol Clin. 2018;7(3):355–65. https://doi.org/10.1016/j.iccl.2018.03.005.. Epub 2018 Jun 29. Review.

12. Gebker R, Jahnke C, Manka R, Hamdan A, Schnackenburg B, Fleck E, Paetsch I. Additional value of myocardial perfusion imaging during dobutamine stress magnetic resonance for the assessment of coronary artery disease. Circ Cardiovasc Imaging. 2008;1(2):122–30. https://doi.org/10.1161/CIRCIMAGING.108.779108.

13. Manka R, Jahnke C, Gebker R, Schnackenburg B, Paetsch I. Head-to-head comparison of first-pass MR perfusion imaging during adenosine and high-dose dobutamine/atropine stress. Int J Cardiovasc Imaging. 2011;27(7):995–1002. https://doi.org/10.1007/s10554-010-9748-3.

14. Morton G, Schuster A, Perera D, Nagel E. Cardiac magnetic resonance imaging to guide complex revascularization in stable coronary artery disease. Eur Heart J. 2010;31(18):2209–15. https://doi.org/10.1093/eurheartj/ehq256.

15. Wellnhofer E, Olariu A, Klein C, Gräfe M, Wahl A, Fleck E, Nagel E. Magnetic resonance low-dose dobutamine test is superior to SCAR quantification for the prediction of functional recovery. Circulation. 2004;109(18):2172–4.. Epub 2004 Apr 26.

Valvular Heart Diseases

4

4.1 Mitral Valve

4.1.1 Degenerative Mitral and Aortic Valvulopathy

Medical History Male, 68 y.o. Dyspnea on effort. At Echocardiography evidence of aortic and mitral degenerative disease.

CMR Flowchart Stack of cine images in short-axis view to evaluate biventricular volumes, function, and segmental thickness. Cine images in short axis of the aortic valve to measure residual opening. Cine images in long axes of the heart (vertical and horizontal) to evaluate mitral opening.

Postcontrast LGE to assess the presence of intramyocardial fibrosis.

Main CMR Findings Left-ventricle volume and global function normal. Diffuse wall hypertrophy (max thickness at the level of the interventricular septum: 14 mm). Residual opening area of the aortic valve: 0.85 cm^2. Light aortic regurgitation (regurgitant fraction 10%). Thickened mitral valve leaflets with reduced diastolic opening. No intramyocardial fibrosis. Left atrium enlargement (Movie 4.1, Movie 4.2 and Movie 4.3).

Conclusion Degenerative valvular disease involving both the mitral (stenosis) and the aortic valve (stenosis and regurgitation).

Electronic Supplementary Material The online version of this chapter (https://doi.org/10.1007/978-3-030-41830-4_4) contains supplementary material, which is available to authorized users.

© Springer Nature Switzerland AG 2020
Y. Rustamova, M. Lombardi, *Cardiac Magnetic Resonance Atlas*, https://doi.org/10.1007/978-3-030-41830-4_4

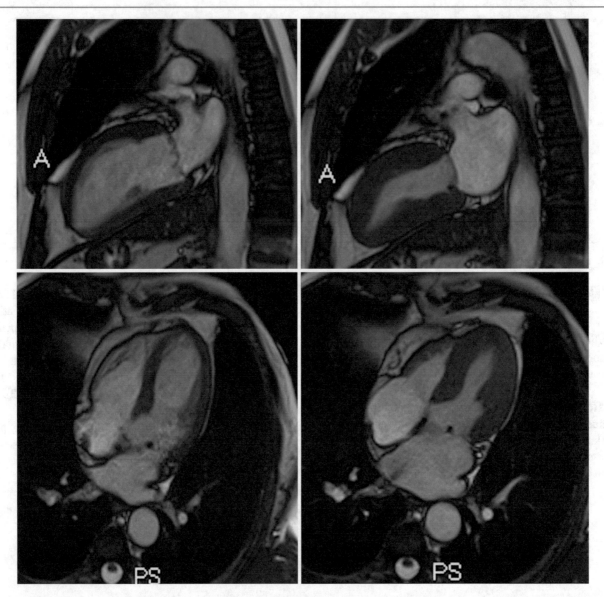

Fig. 4.1 SSFP cine images in vertical long-axis (upper panels) and horizontal long-axis (lower panels) views. Diffuse hypertrophy in the presence of normal function. Left panels: diastolic frames; right panels: systolic frames

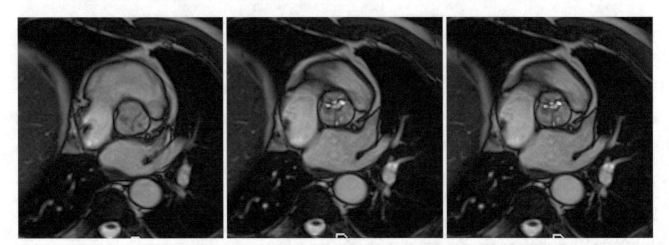

Fig. 4.2 SSFP cine images in short axis of the aortic valve. Evidence of thickened valvular leaflets. The planimetric measurement showed a residual 0.85 cm² systolic opening. Left panel: diastolic phase. Mid panel: systolic phase. Right panel: planimetric measurement of residual area during the systolic phase

4.1.2 Mitral Prolapse

Medical History Female, 61 y.o. Palpitation.

CMR Flowchart Stack of cine images in short-axis view to evaluate biventricular volumes and function. Cine images in vertical and horizontal long axis to evaluate the mitral valve movement. LGE images to evaluate the presence of intramyocardial fibrosis.

Main CMR Findings Normal biventricular regional and global function. At cine images presence of severe prolapse of both the mitral leaflets. Evidence of severe mitral regurgitation. At LGE images evidence of intramyocardial fibrosis at the level of the posterior leaflet implant (Movie 4.4 and Movie 4.5).

Conclusion Mitral prolapse with severe valvular regurgitation and intramyocardial fibrosis.

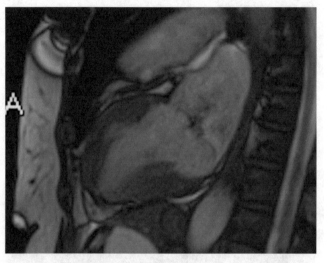

Fig. 4.3 SSFP cine image (still frame) in vertical long-axis plane, end-systolic phase. Evidence of mitral prolapse and mitral regurgitation

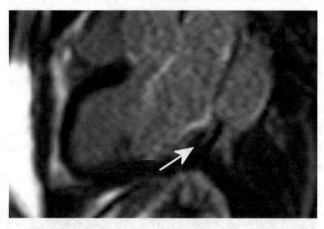

Fig. 4.5 LGE image. Vertical long-axis view. The arrow shows the intramyocardial fibrosis at the level of the posterior mitral leaflet implant

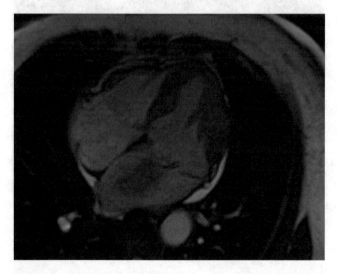

Fig. 4.4 SSFP cine image (still frame) in horizontal long-axis plane, end-systolic phase. Evidence of mitral prolapse and mitral regurgitation

4.1.3   Previous Valvuloplasty in Rheumatic Mitral Valve

Clinical History Seventy-one-year-old female patient with permanent atrial fibrillation. Twenty years earlier she underwent mitral commissurotomy and valvular annuloplasty (Gore-Tex) because of a severe post-rheumatic valvulopathy. She received also a tricuspid annuloplasty and aortic valvuloplasty. Subsequent development of dilatative cardiomyopathy within normal coronary arteries.

At echocardiographic examination, 1 year earlier, a severe dilatation of the left atrium was reported, a spherically enlarged left ventricle with the reduced ejection fraction (LVEF = 35%), moderate-to-severe mitral regurgitation, mild aortic regurgitation, moderate tricuspid regurgitation with slightly elevated pulmonary artery pressure (35 mm Hg).

Patient symptomatic for dyspnea on exertion.

CMR Flowchart Cine images in vertical and horizontal long axis. Stack of cine images in short axis of the left ventricle to evaluate biventricular volumes and function. T2w images to exclude inflammatory processes. LGE images to exclude fibronecrotic areas within the myocardium. Phase-contrast images were not collected because of atrial fibrillation.

Main CMR Findings Eccentric myocardial hypertrophy with moderate-to-severe left ventricular dysfunction (LVEF = 35%) with global hypokinesis. Severe dilatation of left atrium (Movie 4.6).

Right ventricle's size and volumes are within normal range with the ejection fraction at lower limits of normality (RVEF = 45%) (Movie 4.7).

Moderate mitral regurgitation (qualitative evaluation), moderate aortic regurgitation, mild tricuspid regurgitation (Movie 4.8).

Conclusion Cardiopathy on rheumatic valvular pathology basis.

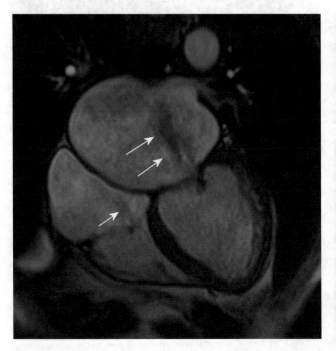

Fig. 4.6 SSFP cine images in horizontal long axis. Mid-systolic frame. The arrows show the turbulence due to mitral and tricuspid regurgitation

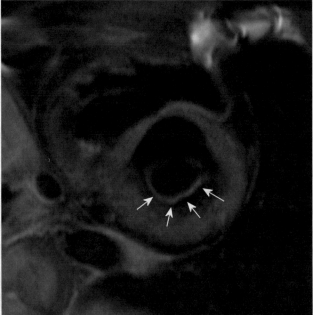

Fig. 4.7 T2w images in short axis of left ventricle. The arrows show the Gore-Tex annulus used for the mitral valvuloplasty

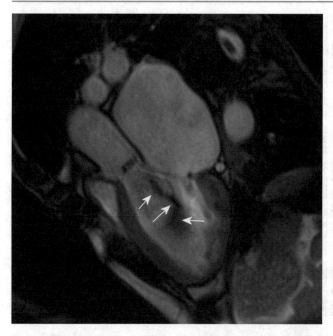

Fig. 4.8 SSFP cine images in three-chamber view. Diastolic frame. The arrows show the turbulence due to the severe aortic valve regurgitation

4.1.4 Parachute Mitral Valve

Medical History Female, 8 y.o. Asymptomatic. Congenital heart disease: Interventricular defect (previously surgically corrected), bicuspid aortic valve, parachute mitral valve, aortic coartation (previously surgically corrected).

CMR Flowchart Stack of cine images in short-axis view to evaluate biventricular volumes and function. Cine images in oblique view to obtain diagnostic images at the level of the single papillary muscle. Images in short-axis view of the aortic valve. Cine images of the thoracic aorta ("candy-cane" view). Phase-contrast images at the level of the aortic valve. Contrast-Enhanced Magnetic Resonance Angiography (CEMRA) of the thoracic aorta.

Main CMR Findings Left-ventricle volume and global function normal. Presence of a single papillary muscle connected to both mitral valve leaflets (Movie 4.9 and Movie 4.10). Presence of bicuspid aortic valve with two Valsalva sinuses (Movie 4.11). Normal function either of the mitral valve or of the aortic valve. No evidence of aortic coartation.

Conclusion Parachute mitral valve and bicuspid aortic valve.

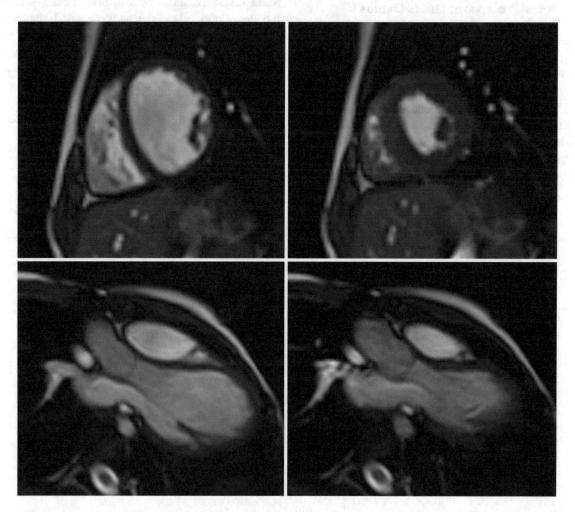

Fig. 4.9 SSFP cine images in short-axis (upper panels) and three-chamber views (lower panels) in end diastole (left panels) and end systole (right panels). Evidence of a single papillary muscle

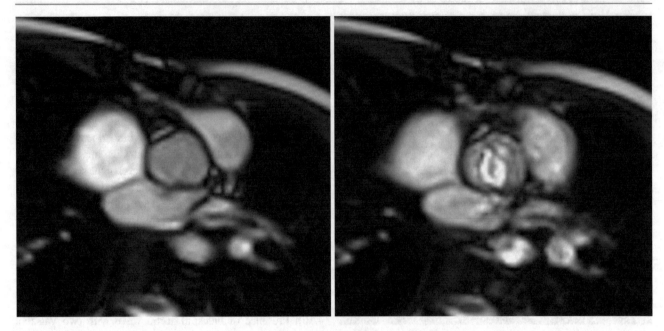

Fig. 4.10 SSFP cine images in short axis of the aortic valve. Evidence of two Valsalva sinuses and bicuspid opening. Left panel: end-diastolic frame; right panel: end-systolic frame

4.1.5   Mitral Prolapse in Ehlers-Danlos Syndrome

Medical History   Previous diagnosis of Ehlers-Danlos syndrome. Palpitation and dyspnea.

CMR Flowchart   Stack of cine images in short-axis view to evaluate biventricular volumes and function. SSFP cine images in horizontal long-axis planes to evaluate the mitral valve. Cine images in oblique view (sagittal) to assess the thoracic aorta. LGE images to detect myocardial fibrosis.

Main CMR Findings   Normal biventricular volumes and function. Normal dimension and course of the thoracic aorta. Evidence of prolapsing mitral anterior leaflet. No evidence of mitral regurgitation (Movie 4.12). No myocardial fibrosis at LGE images. Normal course and diameters of thoracic Aorta (Movie 4.13).

Conclusion   Mitral prolapse in Ehlers-Danlos syndrome.

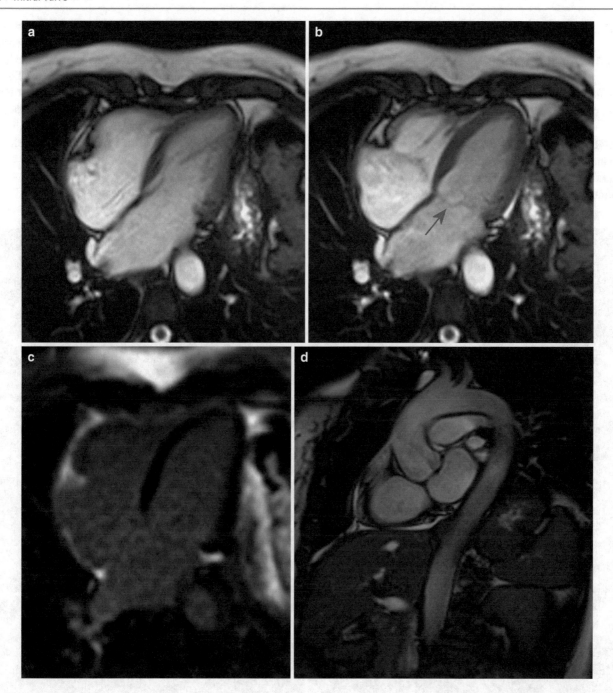

Fig. 4.11 Panel **a**: SSFP cine image in horizontal long axis, end-diastolic frame. Panel **b**: SSFP cine image in horizontal long axis, end-systolic frame. The red arrow shows the anterior leaflet prolapse. Panel **c**: LGE image in horizontal long axis; no evidence of myocardial fibro-sis. Panel **d**: SSFP cine images in sagittal plane to assess the morphology of thoracic aorta which shows a normal course and normal diameters

4.2 Aortic Valve

4.2.1 Aortic Stenosis

Medical History Patient with renal failure treated regularly with dialysis. Severe aortic stenosis at Echocardiography.

CMR Flowchart Stack of cine images in short-axis view to evaluate biventricular volumes and function and to assess wall thickness and ventricular mass. Stack of cine images in oblique plane and short axis of the aortic valve. LGE images.

Main CMR Findings Diffuse increase of left-ventricle wall thickness. Left-ventricle volumes and function within the limits. Dilated left atrium. Turbulence of flow at the level of the aortic valve and ascending aorta which is slightly dilated (Movie 4.14 and Movie 4.15). Gross morphologic abnormalities of the aortic leaflets with a moderate reduction of the planimetric area (1.42 cm²) (Movie 4.16). Increase of flow speed at the level of the aortic valve with a max velocity of 470 cm/s.

Conclusion Degenerative aortic stenosis.

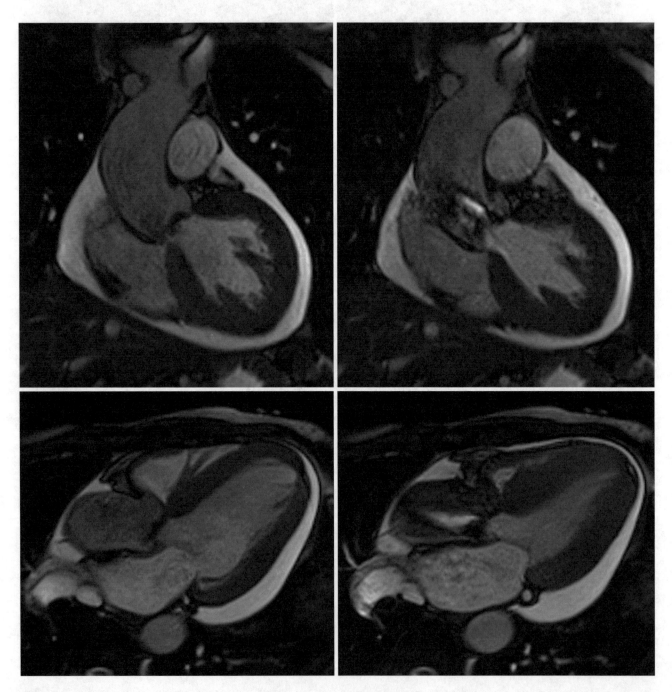

Fig. 4.12 Stack of SSFP cine images in coronal plane (upper panels) and in horizontal long axis of the heart (lower panels). Evidence of gross morphologic abnormalities of the aortic leaflets during the dia-stolic phase (left panels) and turbulence of flow during the systolic phase (right panels). Presence of a moderate pericardial effusion

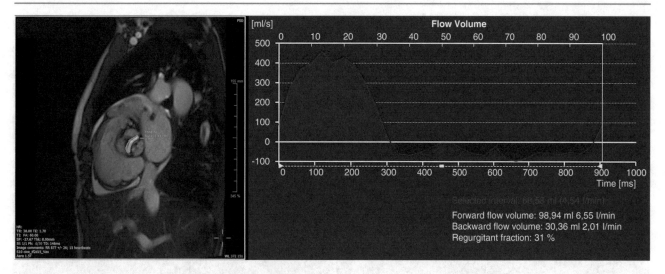

Fig. 4.13 Left panel: morphologic image of the aortic valve (SPSS cine image, systolic phase). The planimetric measurement reveals a moderate reduction of the residual area (1.42 cm²). Right panel: results of the post-processing analysis of the flow sequence. Evidence of significant increase of the systolic flow velocity (max 470 cm/s). Furthermore the analysis reveals a moderate aortic regurgitation

4.2.2   Aortic Valve Regurgitation

Medical History   Male, 17 y.o. Suspected previous episode of rheumatic fever. Evidence at Echocardiography of aortic regurgitation and at last visit doubtful enlargement of left ventricle with preserved global function.

CMR Flowchart   Stack of cine images in short-axis view to evaluate biventricular volumes and function. Cine images in short axis of the aortic valve to evaluate valvular morphology and motion. Phase-contrast images at the level of aortic valve and at the level of pulmonary valve to evaluate the regurgitation fraction. 3D angiography (CEMRA) to evaluate the aortic course and morphology. LGE images to detect eventual myocardial fibrosis.

Main CMR Findings   Left ventricular enlargement (110 ml/m²) with preserved global function (EF 65%) (Movie 4.17). Aortic valve with three Valsalva sinuses. Morphologically abnormal aortic valve, whose leaflets appear thickened but with normal systolic/diastolic movement. Moderate/severe aortic regurgitation (regurgitant fraction 40%) (Movie 4.18 and Movie 4.19). No aortic dilatation. No intramyocardial fibrosis at LGE images.

Conclusion   Initial left-ventricle dilatation in a patient with moderate-severe aortic regurgitation probably due to previous rheumatic infection.

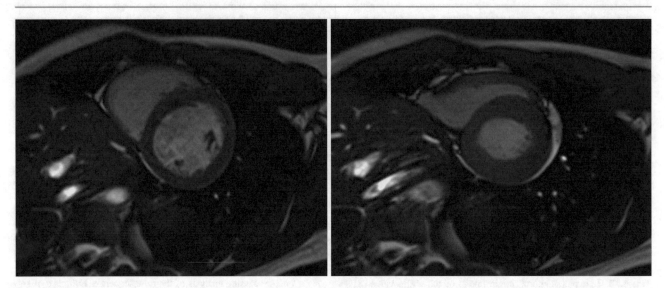

Fig. 4.14 Cine images. End-diastolic (left panel) and end-systolic (right panel) frames. Initial dilatation of the left ventricle with normal global function

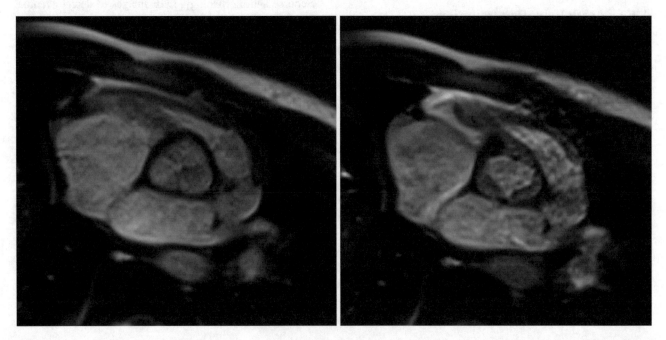

Fig. 4.15 Cine images. End-diastolic (left panel) and end-systolic (right panel) frames. Aortic valve thickened with lack of coaptation during the diastole

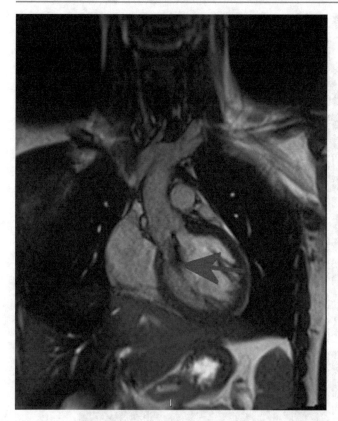

Fig. 4.16 Cine frame in early diastole. Evidence of significant regurgitation (arrow)

Fig. 4.17 Resulting scheme of transvalvular flow computed on phase-contrast images. At the end of the systolic phase there is a backward flow lasting for the whole diastolic phase which represents 40% of the total flow

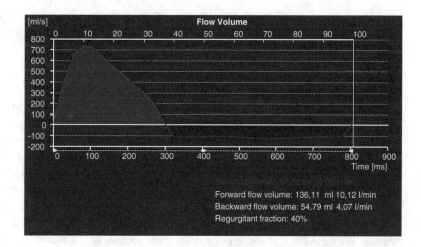

4.2.3 Aortic Subvalvular Stenosis

Medical History Female, 22 y.o. Affected by rheumatoid arthritis. Chest pain and dyspnea. Subvalvular aortic stenosis (trans-stenotic gradient evaluated by Doppler Echocardiography: 42 mmHg). Left-ventricle hypertrophy.

CMR Flowchart Stack of cine images in short-axis view to evaluate biventricular volumes and function, wall thickness, and left-ventricle mass. Stack of cine images in oblique plane at the level of the Aortic root to evaluate the aortic valve. LGE images.

Main CMR Findings Concentric left-ventricle hypertrophy. Evidence of turbulent flow at the level of the left-ventricle outflow tract starting about 1 cm below the valvular plane where a tiny linear structure is detectable (Movie 4.20 and Movie 4.21).

Conclusion Subvalvular aortic stenosis due to the presence of a thin membrane-like structure.

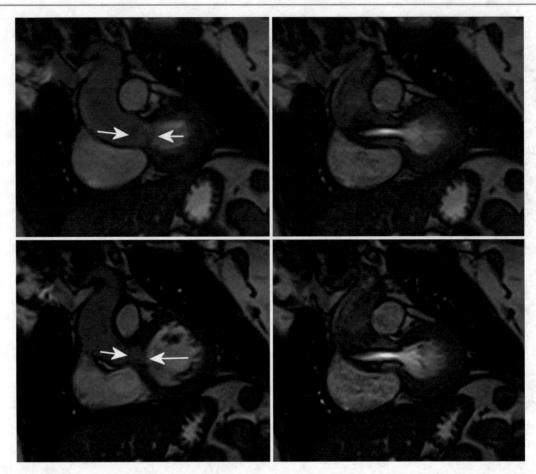

Fig. 4.18 SSFP cine images from two oblique views, in diastole (left panels) and during the ventricular systole (right panels). Evidence of a linear thin structure (left-oriented arrows) 1 cm below the valvular plane (right-oriented arrows). During the systolic phase (right panels) evidence of turbulent flow originating at the level of the subvalvular stenosis

4.2.4 Aortic Subvalvular Stenosis with Valvular Regurgitation

Medical History Male, 54 y.o. Systolic murmur. At Echocardiography evidence of turbulent flow at the level of the left-ventricle outflow tract.

CMR Flowchart Stack of cine images in short-axis view to evaluate biventricular volumes and function. Cine images in oblique view to obtain diagnostic images at the level of the left-ventricle outflow tract. To improve the temporal resolution it is suggested to increase the number of reconstruction phases/heartbeat.

Main CMR Findings Left-ventricle volume and global function normal. In oblique view, the cine images, obtained with a high temporal resolution (100 frames/heartbeat), show the presence of a discrete subaortic membrane, a thickened aortic valve, evidence of turbulent flow at the level of the aortic root and ascending aorta, and evidence of aortic regurgitation (Movie 4.22).

Conclusion Aortic subvalvular stenosis.

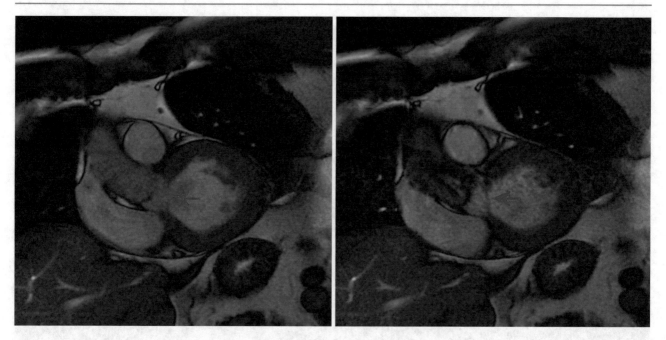

Fig. 4.19 SSFP cine images in oblique view. High-temporal-resolution sequence (100 frames/heartbeat). Left panel: end-diastolic frame. Right panel: end-systolic frame. The arrows show the presence of a discrete subaortic membrane

4.2.5 Bicuspid Aortic Valve

4.2.5.1 Three Valsalva Sinuses and Functional Bicuspid Aortic Valve (BAV)

Medical History Female, 42 y.o. Echocardiographic evidence of bicuspid aortic valve.

CMR Flowchart Stack of cine images in short-axis view to evaluate biventricular volumes, function, and stroke volumes. SSFP cine images in short axis of the aortic valve to evaluate the morphology and the function of the valve. SSSFP cine images to evaluate the ascending aorta, the aortic arch, and the descending thoracic aorta, to evaluate the segmental dimension of the vessel. Contrast-enhanced 3D angiography (CEMRA) to evaluate the three-dimensional morphology of the thoracic aorta. Phase-contrast images at the level of the aortic valve to quantitatively evaluate the aortic regurgitation.

Main CMR Findings Increased volumes of left ventricle (end-diastolic volume: 123 ml/m², end-systolic volume 54 ml/m²). Aortic valve with three Valsalva sinuses and bicuspid function (Movie 4.23). Moderate aortic regurgitation (31%) (Movie 4.24). Ascending aorta dilatation (40 mm) (Movie 4.25).

Conclusion Functionally bicuspid aortic valve opening in the presence of three Valsalva sinuses. Moderate aortic regurgitation in the presence of left-ventricle enlargement and ascending aorta dilatation.

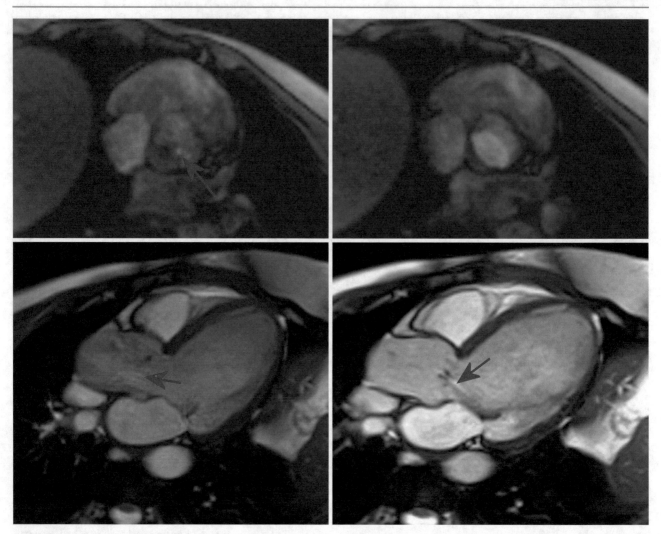

Fig. 4.20 SSFP cine images in short axis of the aortic valve (upper panels), and three-chamber view (lower panels). In end diastole (upper left panel) evidence of lack of coaptation of the valvular leaflets. During the systolic phase (upper right panel) "classical" oval shape of leaflet opening. In three-chamber view, during the systolic phase (lower left panel), evidence of turbulent flow (arrow). During the diastolic phase (lower right panel) evidence of aortic regurgitation (arrow)

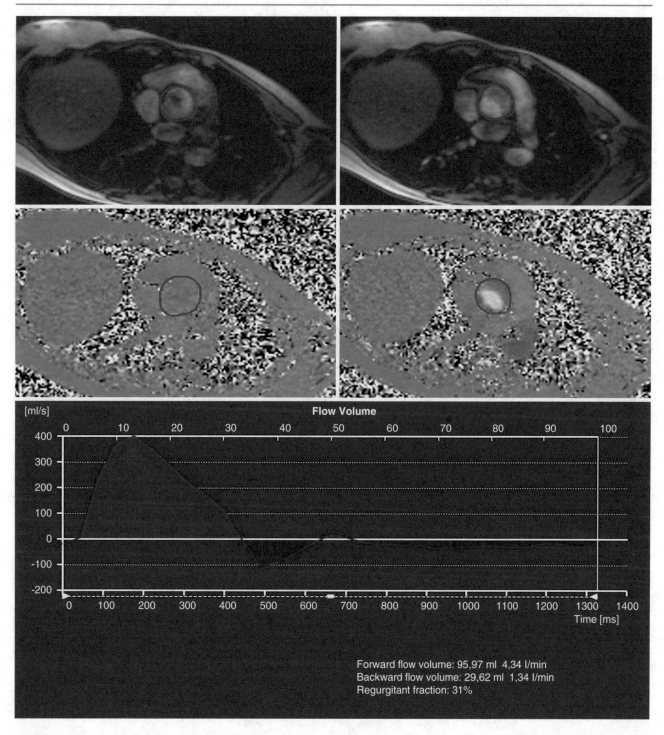

Fig. 4.21 Phase-contrast images to evaluate transvalvular aortic flow. Upper panels: SPSS images of the aortic valve in short-axis view (left panel in end diastole, right panel in end systole). In middle panels the corresponding phase-contrast images to evaluate the transvalvular flow within a region of interest (ROI) manually drawn at the level of the valve (in red). In the lower panel the resulting flow analysis

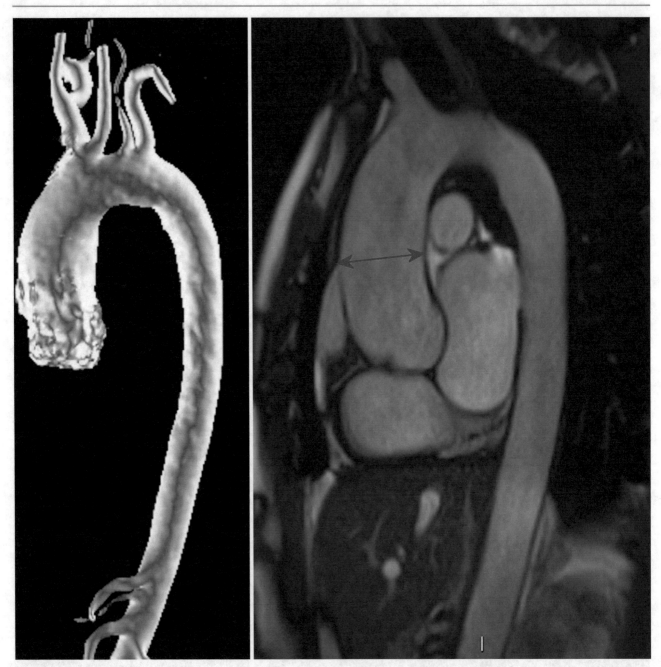

Fig. 4.22 Left panel: three-dimensional contrast-enhanced angiography (CEMRA) and SSFP cine images in paraxial plane to evaluate course and dimension of aorta ("candy-cane" images). Evidence of ascending aorta enlargement (42 mm in anteroposterior direction, comprehensive of the aortic wall thickness). Measurements performed in end systole

4.2.6   Bicuspid Aortic Valve with Two Valsalva Sinuses

Medical History Male, 38 y.o. Asymptomatic. At Echocardiography evidence of abnormal opening of the aortic valve, suspected Bicuspid aortic valve (BAV).

CMR Flowchart Stack of cine images in short-axis view to evaluate biventricular volumes and function. Cine images in oblique short-axis view of the aortic valve. Phase-contrast images at the level of the aortic valve. Cine images of the thoracic aorta ("candy-cane" view). Contrast-enhanced mag-

netic resonance angiography (0.15 mmol/kg). 3D free breathing coronary angiography to exclude coronary artery anomalies of origin and proximal course.

Main CMR Findings Normal biventricular volumes and function. Aortic valve with two Valsalva sinuses (Movie 4.26). Coronary arteries origin from the anterior Valsalva sinus. Normal shape and dimension of the thoracic aorta. Very light aortic regurgitation (Regurgitant Fraction: 6%).

Conclusion Two Valsalva sinuses and bicuspid aortic valve. Origin of Coronary Arteries from the anterior Valsalva Sinus.

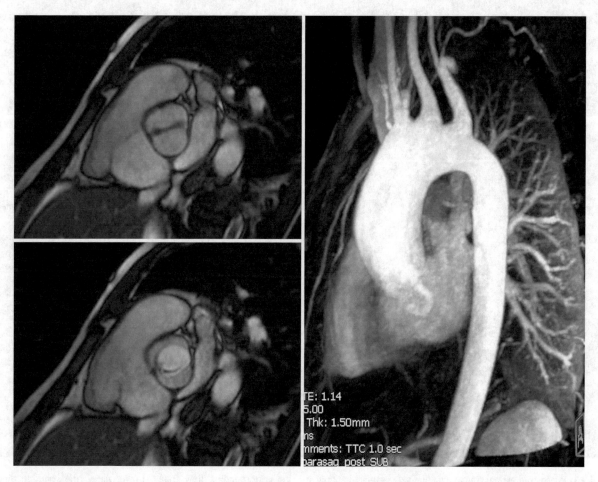

Fig. 4.23 Upper left panel: SSFP cine image in short-axis view of aortic valve. In the end-diastolic frame evidence of one central commissure. Lower left panel: SSFP cine image in short-axis view of aortic valve. In the end-systolic frame evidence of elliptical shaped opening of the valve. Right panel: 3D contrast angiography showing an enlarged ascending aorta (maximum diameter: 46 mm)

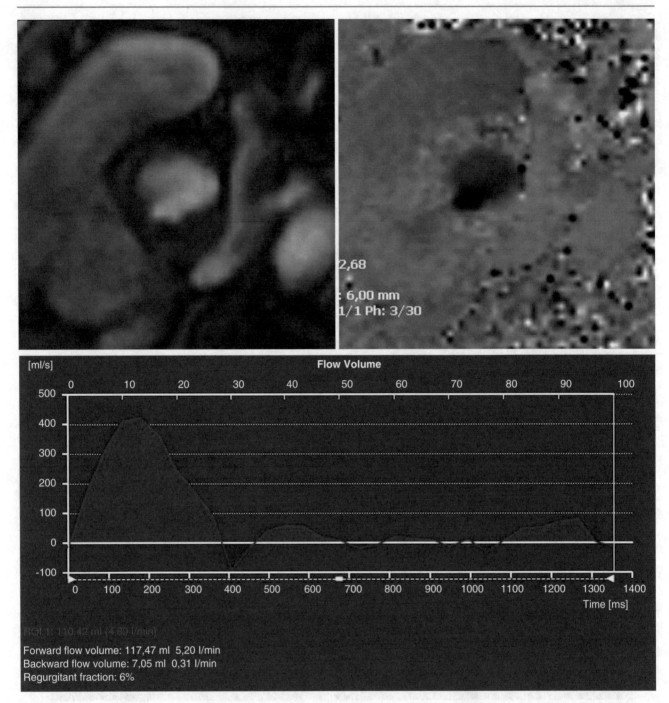

Fig. 4.24 Phase-contrast imaging to quantitatively evaluate the flow at the aortic valve level. Left upper panel: magnitude imaging showing the elliptical shaped end-systolic opening of the valve. Right upper panel: the corresponding flow frame. Lower panel: the resulting diagram showing the quantitative evaluation of forward and backward flow

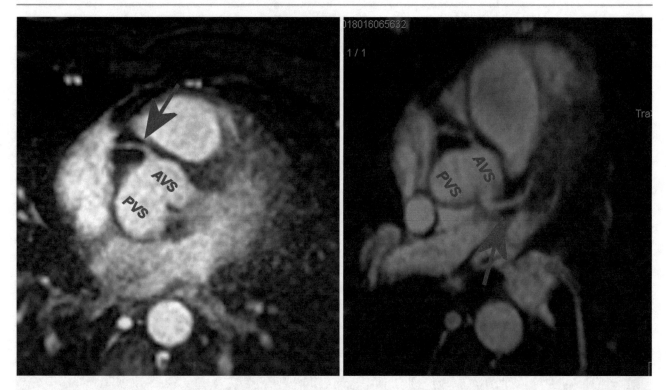

Fig. 4.25 Three-dimensional free-breathing angiography at the level of the coronary artery. Left panel: reconstructed image obtained in a plane to show the origin of the right coronary artery (arrow). Right panel: reconstructed image obtained in a plane to show the origin of the left coronary artery (arrow) (AVS: Anterior Valsalva Sinus; PVS: Posterior Valsalva Sinus)

4.2.7 Bicuspid Aortic Valve Plus Aortic Coartation

Medical History Female, 60 y.o. Systolic murmur. At Echocardiography evidence of turbulent flow at the level of isthmic aorta. Suspect of aortic coarctation.

CMR Flowchart Stack of cine images in short-axis view to evaluate biventricular volumes, global function, and wall thickness. Cine images in oblique view to image the thoracic aorta. Cine images of the aortic valve in short axis. Flow images at the level of the aortic valve, at the level of the ascending aorta, at the level of the aortic arch and immediately before and after the coarctation, and at the level of the diaphragmatic aorta. Contrast-enhanced angio 3D (CEMRA) of thoracic aorta. LGE images.

Main CMR Findings Normal left-ventricle volumes, wall thickness, and global function. Aortic valve with three Valsalva sinuses but with bicuspid behavior (Movie 4.27). Ascending aorta dilatation. Kinking and coarctation at the level of the isthmus (Movie 4.27).

Flow measurement before the origin of Anonymous truncus resulted in 3.74 l/min.

Flow measurement before common left Carotid artery resulted in 2.9 l/min.

Flow measurement immediately after the aortic coarctation resulted in 3.11 l/min.

Flow measurement at the level of the diaphragm resulted in 2.45 l/min.

The residual diameter at the level of the coarctation resulted in 15 mm.

Conclusion Bicuspid morphology of the aortic valve. Aortic coarctation with little hemodynamic consequences.

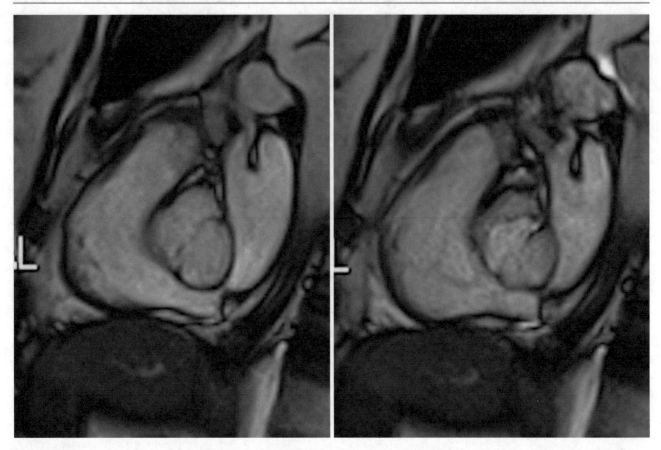

Fig. 4.26 SSFP cine images in short axis of the aortic valve. Left panel: end-diastolic frame. Right panel: end-systolic frame showing the "classical" opening resembling the mouth of a fish of the bicuspid valve

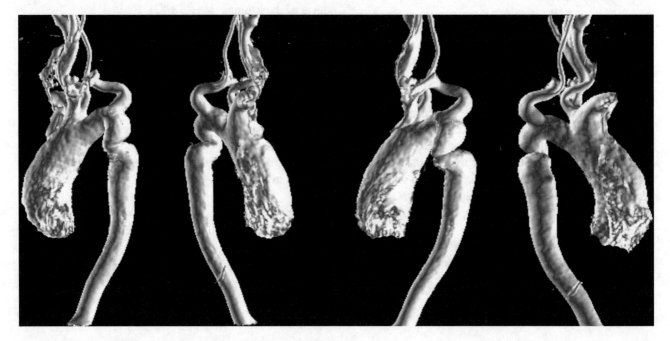

Fig. 4.27 Contrast-enhanced magnetic resonance angiography (CEMRA). The figure shows four angles of view of the thoracic aorta. Evidence of isthmic coarctation

4.3   Tricuspid Valve

4.3.1   Tricuspid Dysplasia

Medical History   Male, 58 y.o. overweight (125 kg, BSA 2.4 m2). Worsening dyspnea. Enlargement of right ventricle at Echocardiography.

CMR Flowchart   Stack of SSFP cine images in short-axis view to evaluate biventricular volumes and function. SSFP cine images in vertical long axis of the right ventricle.

Flow images at the level of ascending Aorta and Pulmonary Artery to evaluate the Qp/Qs.

Main CMR Findings   Normal left-ventricle volumes (EDV 58 ml/m^2, ESV 18 ml/m^2) and function (EF 69%). Abnormal volume of right ventricle (EDV 110 ml/m^2; ESV 51 ml/m^2) with preserved global function (EF 54%). Displacement of tricuspid septal leaflet (21 mm, n.v. <8.8 mm/m^2). Significant tricuspid regurgitation (Movie 4.28, Movie 4.29 and Movie 4.30).

Conclusion   Isolated tricuspid dysplasia.

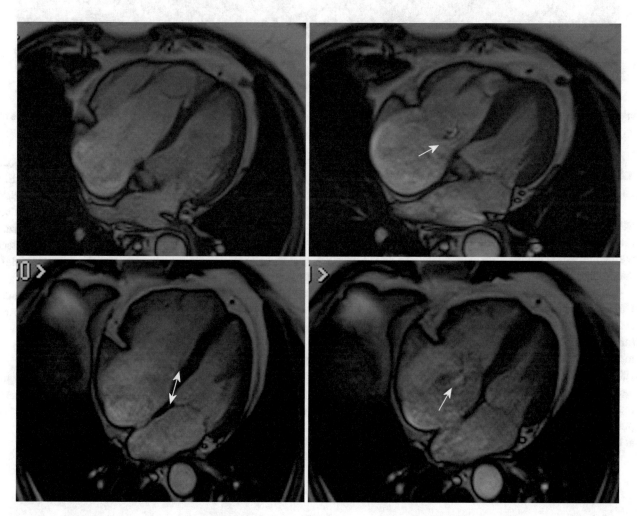

Fig. 4.28   SSFP cine images in two parallel axial planes to evaluate the morphology and function of tricuspid valve. Left panels: diastolic phase. Right panels: systolic phase. Evidence of tricuspid regurgitation during the systolic phase (right panels: arrow) and abnormal distance between the tricuspid septal leaflet and the mitral plane (lower left panel, double-end arrow)

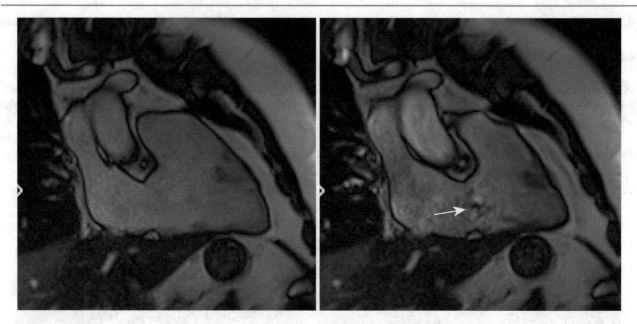

Fig. 4.29 SSFP images in vertical long axis of the right ventricle. Left panel: diastolic phase. During the systolic phase (right panel) evidence of tricuspid regurgitation (arrow)

4.3.2 Ebstein Anomaly of the Tricuspid Valve Disease

Medical History Female, 14 y.o. At the age of 9 years transcatheter closure of ostium secundum atrial septal defects with an umbrella device. Previous pulmonary valvuloplasty due to congenital stenosis. Affected by Ebstein anomaly.

CMR Flowchart Stack of cine images in short-axis view to evaluate biventricular volumes, function, and wall thickness. Stack of horizontal long-axis cine images to evaluate the location of the septal and posterior leaflets of the tricuspid valve and to calculate the percentage of the atrialized right ventricle. Phase-contrast images to quantitatively measure the flow to the level of the ascending aorta, at the level of the pulmonary trunk, at the level of the superior vena cava, and at the level of the subdiaphragmatic aorta.

Main CMR Findings Left-ventricle volume and global function normal. Severe dilatation of right ventricle (ED 190 ml/m^2, ES 81 ml/m^2) with preserved global function (EF 58%). Displacement of the septal leaflet of the tricuspid valve (18 mm/m^2, normal values: <8 mm/m^2) with index of atrialization of 26% (ratio between displacement of the septal leaflets of the tricuspid valve and the long axis of the right ventricle). Severe tricuspid regurgitation (regurgitant fraction 58%). Pulmonary trunk dilatation. Moderate pulmonary regurgitation (regurgitant fraction 38%). Presence of septal occluder (Movie 4.31, Movie 4.32, Movie 4.33 and Movie 4.34).

Conclusion Ebstein anomaly (index of atrialization of 26%). Right-ventricle dilatation. Moderate tricuspid regurgitation. Pulmonary trunk dilatation. Moderate pulmonary regurgitation.

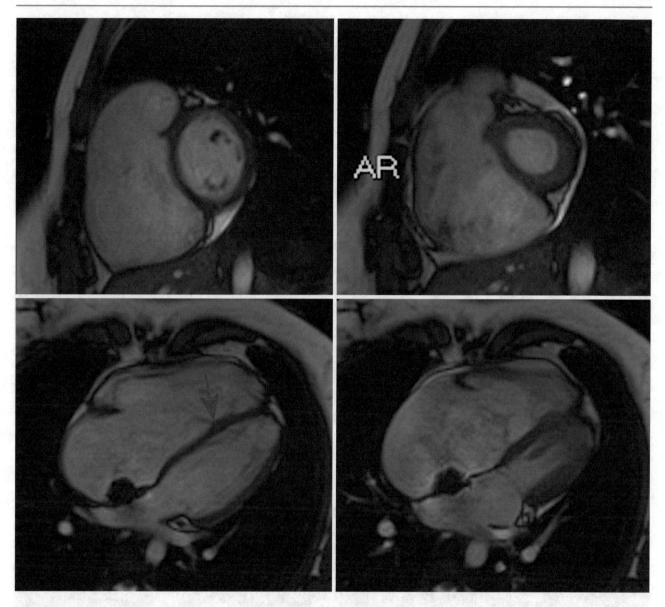

Fig. 4.30   SSFP cine images in short axis (upper panels) and horizontal long axis (lower panels). Left panels: diastolic frames; right panels: systolic frames. Evidence of displacement of the septal leaflets of the tri-cuspid valve (arrow). Right-ventricle enlargement with part of the right ventricle being atrialized. Presence of the atrial septal occluder

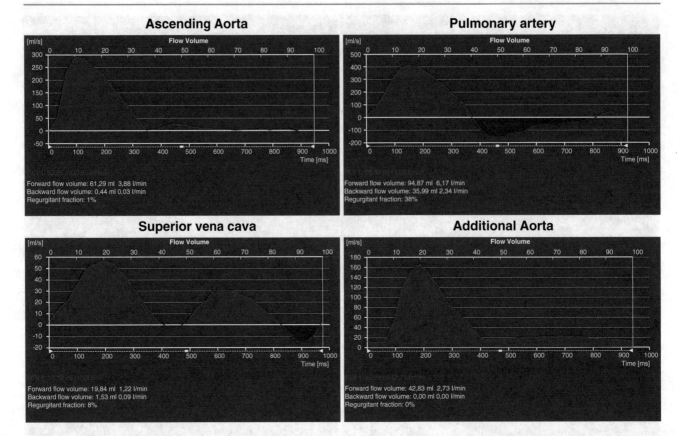

Fig. 4.31 Results of flow measurements at various levels: upper left panel: at the level of the ascending aorta; right upper panel: at the level of the pulmonary trunk; lower left panel: at the level of the superior vena cava; lower right panel: at the level of the subdiaphragmatic aorta to be considered equivalent to the inferior vena cava

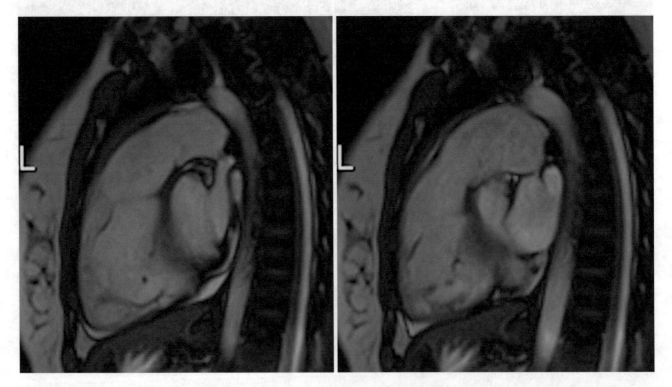

Fig. 4.32 SSFP cine images in oblique plane (parasagittal) to assess the pulmonary trunk which appears to be dilated (left panel: diastolic frame; right panel: systolic frame)

4.4 Pulmonary Valve

4.4.1 Pulmonary Valve Regurgitation, Presurgical Status and Postsurgical Result, Interatrial Defect (Ostium Secundum)

Medical History C.M., female 47 y.o. At the age of 3 years surgical intervention because of a congenital pulmonary valve stenosis. At the age of 46 echocardiographic diagnosis of dilatation of right chambers. In 2017 a CMR was performed to assess the degree of dilatation and the presence of pulmonary regurgitation and to exclude the presence of morphologic abnormalities. In 2018 surgical intervention: positioning of prosthetic valve (Hancock 37) and pericardial patch at the level of the prosthetic pulmonary valve and closure of interatrial defect (ostium secundum).

CMR Flowchart Cine images (SSFP) to evaluate biventricular function, morphology, and dimension of the right-ventricle outflow tract. Cine images to evaluate and also to characterize the interatrial defect. Flow (phase-contrast) images to evaluate the forward flow and to quantitatively evaluate the pulmonary valve regurgitation. Flow images were also collected for a better definition of the interatrial flow. LLGE images were collected to evaluate the presence of intramyocardial fibrosis and the patch position.

Main CMR Findings In the 2017 examination severe right-ventricle dilatation and a severe regurgitation fraction were observed. Furthermore there was an interatrial septal defect (ostium secundum) with Qp/Qs of 1.6 (Movie 4.35, Movie 4.36, Movie 4.37, Movie 4.38, Movie 4.39, Movie 4.40).

In the postsurgical examination (2018) there was a significant reduction of the right-ventricle volume and disappearance of the regurgitation and of the interatrial shunt as well (Movie 4.41, Movie 4.42, Movie 4.43, Movie 4.44, Movie 4.45).

Conclusion Surgical repair of pulmonary regurgitation and of interatrial defect with good final result.

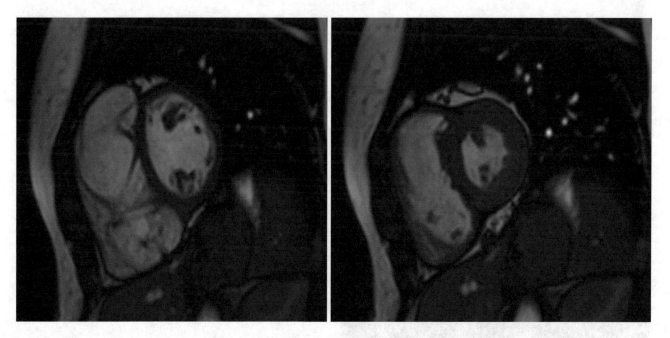

Fig. 4.33 Cine images in short-axis view of the left ventricle. Left panel: diastolic still frame. Right panel: systolic still frame. Significant dilatation of right ventricle

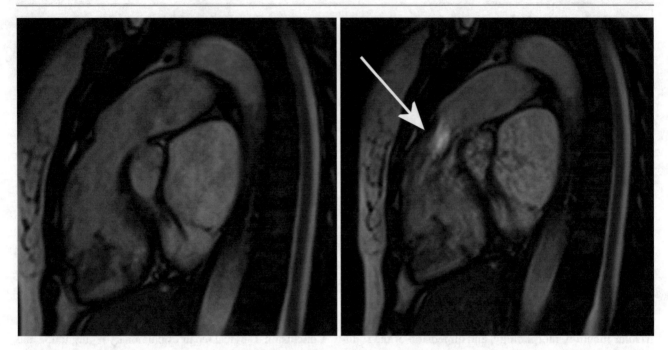

Fig. 4.34 Cine images of right ventricular outflow tract. Left panel: systolic frame. Right panel: protodiastolic frame with evidence of severe regurgitation (arrow)

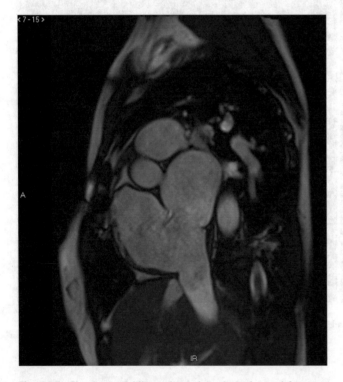

Fig. 4.35 Cine image (oblique plane) through the interatrial septum with evidence of the anatomical defect

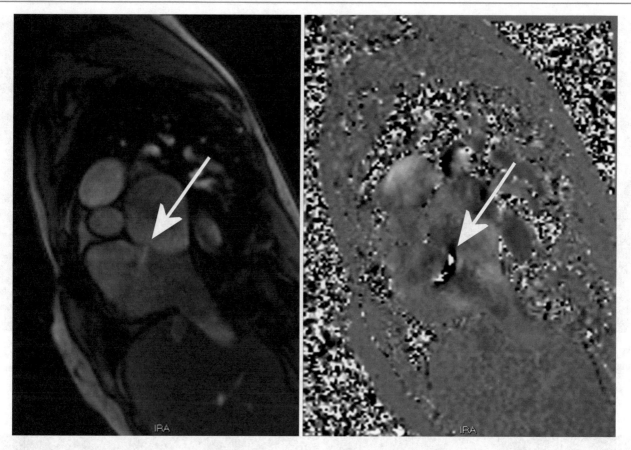

Fig. 4.36 Phase-contrast images of the interatrial defect. Left panel: magnitude image with evidence of flow acceleration (arrow). Right panel: flow image with evidence of aliasing at the same level (arrow)

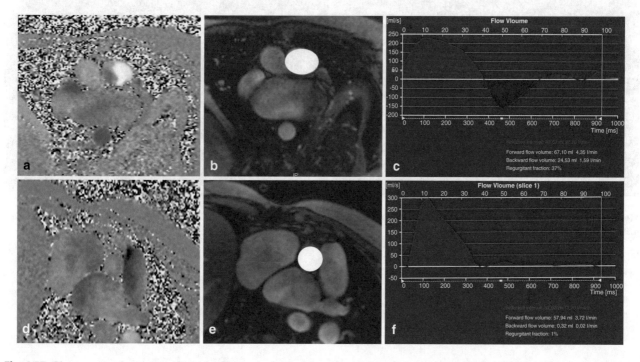

Fig. 4.37 Phase-contrast image to evaluate the flow at the level of the pulmonary trunk (upper panels) and at the level of the ascending aorta (lower panels)

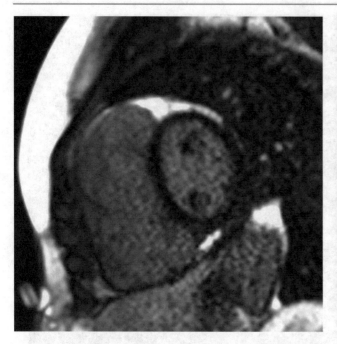

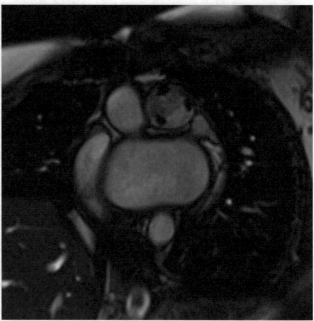

Fig. 4.38 LGE image to exclude the presence of intramyocardial fibrosis. The tiny hyperintensity at the level of the RVOT tract indicates the presence of the surgical patch

Fig. 4.39 Postsurgical image at the level of the pulmonary valve (short axis of the pulmonary trunk just above the valve). Evidence of the three metallic pillars of the valve

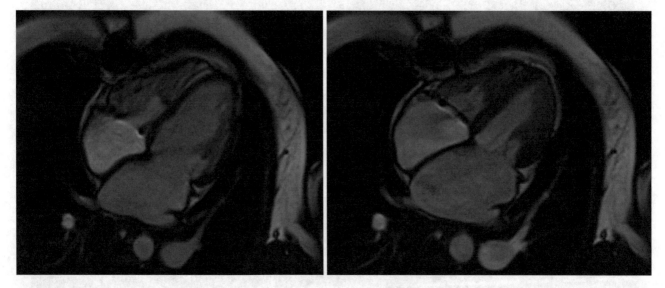

Fig. 4.40 Postsurgical cine images in horizontal long axis of the heart showing a significant reduction of the right-ventricle volumes. Left panel: diastolic frame. Right panel: systolic frame

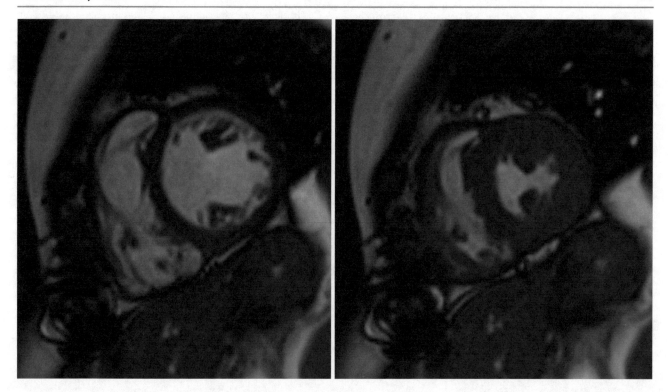

Fig. 4.41 Postsurgical cine images in short axis of the heart showing a significant reduction of the right-ventricle volumes. Left panel: diastolic frame. Right panel: systolic frame

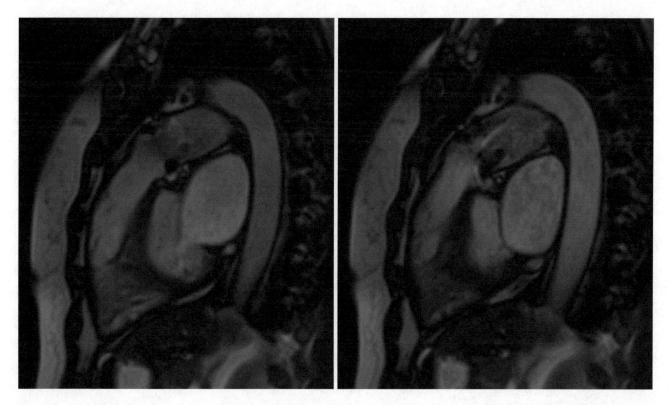

Fig. 4.42 Postsurgical cine images of the right-ventricle outflow tract showing a significant reduction of the right-ventricle volumes. Left panel: diastolic frame. Right panel: systolic frame

Bibliography

1. Lombardi M, Plein S, Petersen S, Bucciarelli-Ducci C, Valsangiacoo Buechel M, Basso C, Ferrari V, editors. The EACVI textbook of cardiovascular magnetic resonance. Oxford: Oxford University Press; 2018.

2. Basso C, Perazzolo Marra M, Rizzo S, De Lazzari M, Giorgi B, Cipriani A, Frigo AC, Rigato I, Migliore F, Pilichou K, Bertaglia E, Cacciavillani L, Bauce B, Corrado D, Thiene G, Iliceto S. Arrhythmic mitral valve prolapse and sudden cardiac death. Circulation. 2015;132:556–66.

3. Marino BS, Kruge LE, Cho CJ, Tomlinson RS, Shera D, Weinberg PM, Gaynor JW, Rychik J. Parachute mitral valve: morphologic descriptors, associated lesions, and outcomes after biventricular repair. J Thorac Cardiovasc Surg. 2009;137(2):385–93.e4.

4. Kawel-Boehm N, Maceira A, Valsangiacomo-Buechel ER, Vogel-Claussen J, Turkbey EB, Williams R, Plein S, Tee M, Eng J, Bluemke DA. Normal values for cardiovascular magnetic resonance in adults and children. J Cardiovasc Magn Reson. 2015;17:29.

5. Wassmuth R, von Knobelsdorff-Brenkenhoff F, Gruettner H, Utz W, Schulz-Menger J. Cardiac magnetic resonance imaging of congenital bicuspid aortic valves and associated aortic pathologies in adults. Eur Heart J Cardiovasc Imaging. 2014;15(6):673–9.

6. Shenoy C, Maron MS, Natesa G. Pandian Cardiovascular magnetic resonance imaging for bicuspid aortic valve syndrome: the time is now. Eur Heart J Cardiovasc Imaging. 2014;15(6):612–4.

7. Opotowsky AR, Pickard SS, Geva T. Imaging adult patients with discrete subvalvular aortic stenosis. Curr Opin Cardiol. 2017;32(5):513–20.

8. Hösch O, Sohns JM, Nguyen TT, Lauerer P, Rosenberg C, Kowallick JT, Kutty S, Unterberg C, Schuster A, Faßhauer M, Staab W, Paul T, Lotz J, Steinmetz M. The total right/left-volume index: a new and simplified cardiac magnetic resonance measure to evaluate the severity of Ebstein anomaly of the tricuspid valve: a comparison with heart failure markers from various modalities. Circ Cardiovasc Imaging. 2014;7(4):601–9.

9. Rydman R, Shiina Y, Diller GP, Niwa K, Li W, Uemura H, Uebing A, Barbero U, Bouzas B, Ernst S, Wong T, Pennell DJ, Gatzoulis MA, Babu-Narayan SV. Major adverse events and atrial tachycardia in Ebstein's anomaly predicted by cardiovascular magnetic resonance. Heart. 2018;104(1):37–44.

10. Rutz T, Kühn A. The challenge of risk stratification in Ebstein's anomaly. Int J Cardiol. 2019;278:89–90.

Cardiac Masses

5.1 Benign Tumors

5.1.1 Myxoma

Medical History Male, 73 y.o. Evidence at Echocardiography of an intra-atrial mass. Asymptomatic.

CMR Flowchart Stack of cine images in short-axis view to evaluate biventricular volumes and function. Cine images in oblique view to detect the presence, dimension, and shape of the intra-atrial mass. The mobility and the hemodynamic influence are also worth of evaluation. Images in T1w and T2w to evaluate the signal behavior of the mass. First-pass images to evaluate the vascularization of the mass. LGE images to evaluate the fibrotic component of the mass.

Main CMR Findings Normal biventricular volumes and global function. Presence of a small ($15 * 10 * 10$ mm (AP $*$ LL $*$ SI)) round-shaped mass at the level of the interatrial septum, within the left atrial cavity (Movie 5.1). The mass neither shows an infiltrative behavior nor influences the hemodynamic conditions. The mass appears to have a high intensity albeit dis-homogeneous signal in T2 images, isointensity with respect to the myocardium in T1w image. The first-pass images show a good vascularization and LGE images a dis-homogeneous uptake of the contrast agent.

Conclusion Intra-atrial myxoma.

Electronic Supplementary Material The online version of this chapter (https://doi.org/10.1007/978-3-030-41830-4_5) contains supplementary material, which is available to authorized users.

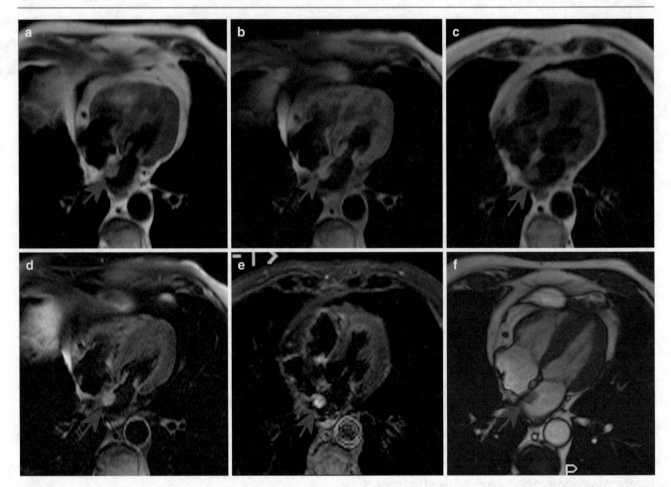

Fig. 5.1 (a) PDw image showing a slight hyperintensity of the mass. (b) T1w fat-saturated image showing isointensity of the mass. (c) T1w image showing isointensity of the mass. (d) T2w SPAIR image showing hyperintensity of the mass. T2w STIR image showing hyperintensity of the mass. SSFP cine image (systolic frame). The arrows show the intra-atrial mass

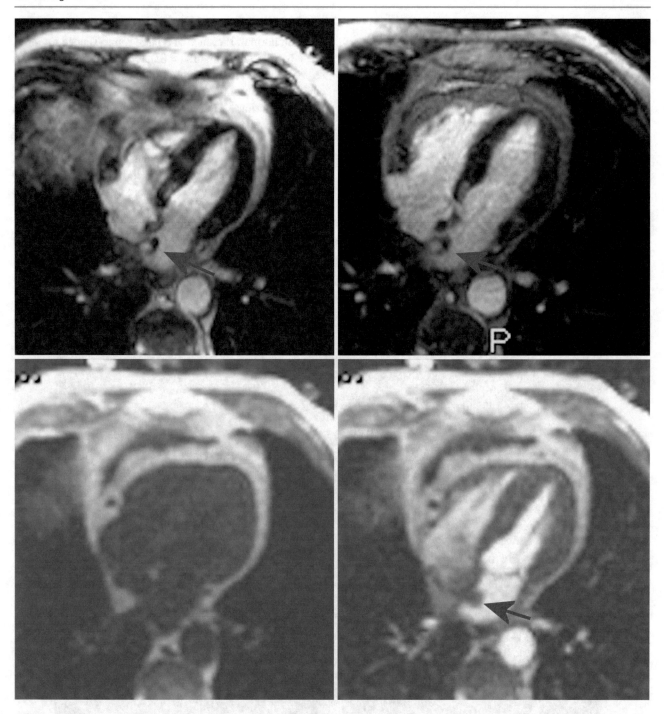

Fig. 5.2 Upper panels: LGE images of two parallel slices of the heart in horizontal long axis. The arrows show a dis-homogeneous uptake of the c.a. Lower panels: two images from a first-pass sequence. Left lower panel: before the contrast agent passes. Right lower panel: during the first pass. Evidence of a perfusion level equivalent to the one of the myocardium

5.1.2   Fibroma

Medical History Male, 15 y.o. Echocardiographic diagnosis of cardiac mass at the age of 1. Diagnosis confirmed at the age of 6 by a Cardiac Magnetic Resonance study.

CMR Flowchart Stack of cine images in short-axis view to evaluate biventricular volumes and function and to identify the presence and location of the known pathologic mass. Cine images in oblique planes to obtain realistic measurements of the tumor and the eventual hemodynamic interference. T1w, T2w, first-pass images, and LGE images to characterize the tissue component of the tumor.

Main CMR Findings Left-ventricle volume and global function normal. Presence of a large round-shaped tumor of 7.5 ∗ 6 ∗ 5.5 cm (AP ∗ LL ∗ SI) at the level of the inferior segments. The tumor is protruding toward the left-ventricle cavity and the right-ventricle cavity as well. No evidence of infiltrative attitude. Evidence of initial compressive effect on the inferior vena cava. No pleuro-pericardial effusion (Movie 5.2, Movie 5.3, Movie 5.4 and Movie 5.5). The signal characteristic, the first-pass signal enhancement (see Fig. 5.5) (Movie 5.6), and the uptake of the contrast agent (see Fig. 5.6) lead to the diagnosis of scarcely aggressive tumor.

Conclusion Cardiac fibroma.

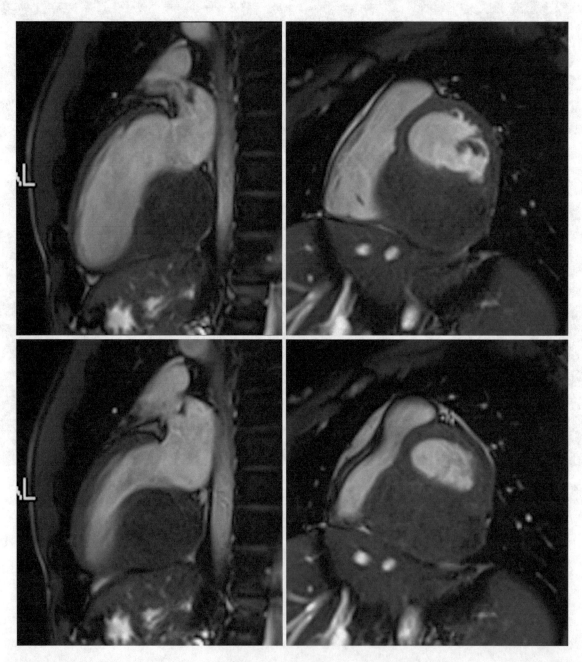

Fig. 5.3 SSFP cine images in vertical long axis (left panels) and in short axis (right panels) of the left ventricle at end diastole (upper panels) and at end systole (lower panels). Evidence of a large round-shaped mass at the level of the inferior and inferoseptal wall which is substituting the myocardial tissue

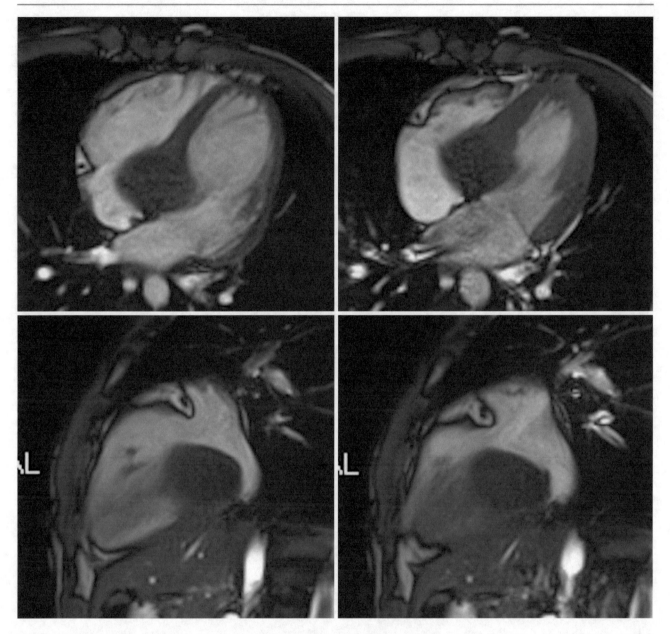

Fig. 5.4 SSFP cine images in horizontal long axis of the heart (upper panels) and vertical long axis of the right sections (lower panels). Images obtained at end diastole (left panels) and end systole (right pan-els). Evidence of a large round-shaped tumor protruding into the left and into the right sections of the heart. Initial compression of inferior vena cava (lower left panel) during the diastolic phase

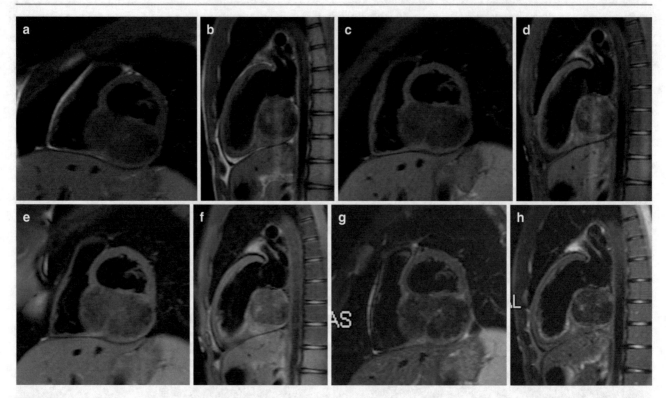

Fig. 5.5 Images obtained with different weighting and with and without fat suppression: (**a** and **b**) proton density weighting (**a** in short axis and **b** in vertical long axis of the left ventricle); (**c** and **d**) proton density weighting and fat saturation (**c** in short axis and **b** in vertical long axis of the left ventricle); (**e** and **f**) T1 weighted (**e** in short axis and **f** in vertical long axis of the left ventricle); (**g** and **h**) STIR T2-weighted images (**g** in short axis and **h** in vertical long axis of the left ventricle)—The tumoral mass shows a large slightly dis-homogeneous hypointense core surrounded by an isointense peripheral layer

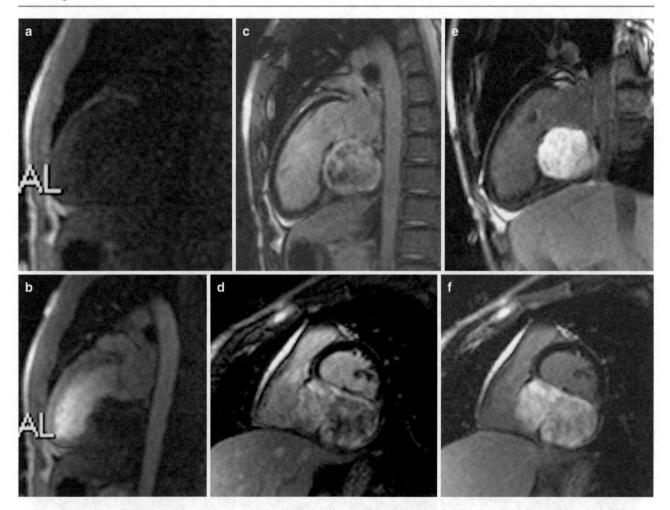

Fig. 5.6 Left panels: first-pass images (**a** before the contrast arrival and **b** during the first pass). Evidence of a reduced signal enhancement during the first pass. GRE-IR images 3 min after the contrast agent injection (0.2 mmol/kg). Evidence of a round-shaped tumor with dishomogeneous uptake of the contrast agent which is more evident on the peripheral layers (**c**: vertical long axis of the left ventricle; **d**: short axis of the heart). Right panels: GRE-IR images (LGE technique) acquired 10 min after the contrast agent injection: evidence of a diffuse uptake of the contrast agent (**e**: vertical long axis of the left ventricle; **f**: short axis of the heart)

5.1.3 Lipoma

Medical History Female, 33 y.o. Dyspnea. Evidence at Echocardiography of an intraventricular mass.

CMR Flowchart Stack of SSFP cine images in short-axis view to evaluate biventricular volumes and function and to assess the presence, location, and extension of the intraventricular mass. SSFP cine images in oblique planes to assess the extension, morphology, and hemodynamic effects of the intracardiac mass. Black blood T1w and T2w images to characterize the mass. Perfusion sequence to evaluate the first pass of a bolus of contrast agent to evaluate the vascularization of the tissue. LGE images.

Main CMR Findings Presence of a round-shaped intraventricular mass (Movie 5.7). The mass is hyperintense in T1w and T2w images while strongly hypointense in images with fat saturaton (STIR). The perfusion images show a low grade of vascularization (Movie 5.8). LGE images show an inhomogeneous uptake of the contrast agent.

Conclusion Intraventricular lipoma with fibrous component.

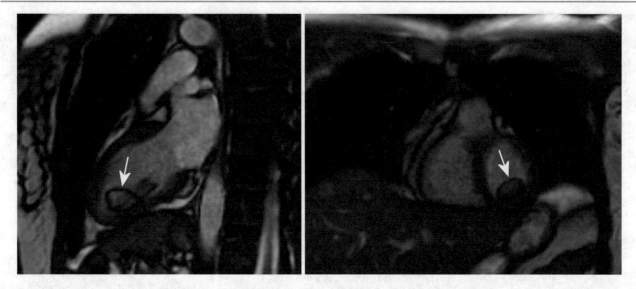

Fig. 5.7 Stack of SSFP cine in vertical long axis (left panel) and short axis of the heart (right panel). The arrows show the presence of a large, sessile, ovoid mass at the level of the inferior wall of the left ventricle. In these images the large black dark rim surrounding the mass is due to the unavoidable chemical shift between the blood and the lipoma

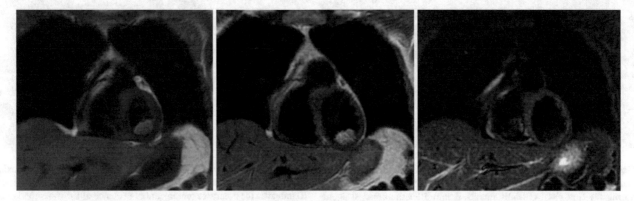

Fig. 5.8 Black blood T1w (left panel), T2w (middle panel), and STIR T2w images (right panel)—The mass appears to be hyperintense in T1w and strongly hyperintense in T2w images while it is completely suppressed in STIR images. Black blood T1-weighted image: TR 722 ms, TE 7 ms. Black blood T2-weighted image: TR 2857 ms, TE 64 ms

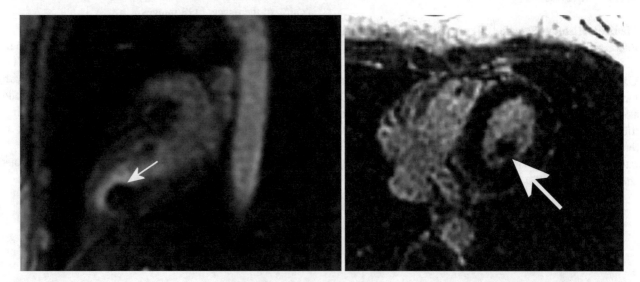

Fig. 5.9 Left panel: single frame from a perfusion sequence obtained during the first pass of a bolus of contrast i.v. injected. Evidence of a dis-homogeneous reduced perfusion at the level of the mass. Right panel: LGE image showing a dis-homogeneous uptake of the c.a. presumably due to the mixture of lipid and fibrotic tissue

5.1.4 Caseous Necrosis

Medical History Female, 77 y.o.

Hypertension. Chronic persistent atrial fibrillation. Presence at Echocardiography, as unexpected finding of a round-shaped mass close to posterior mitral leaflet.

CMR Flowchart Stack of SSFP cine images in short-axis view to evaluate biventricular volumes and function and to assess the presence, location, and extension of the intraventricular mass. Cine images in at least two different projections to evaluate the relationship between the identified mass and the mitral valve. BB T1w images, BB T2w images, eventually BB PDw images. BB T1w postcontrast images, perfusion images, LGE images at the level of the identified mass.

Main CMR Findings Normal bi-ventricular global and regional function. At the level of the inferior wall it is detectable the presence of an ovoid mass, close to the posterior leaflet of the mitral valve (Movie 5.9). No influence on the dynamic movement of the valve. The mass is markedly hypointense in cine images (SSFP), T1w, T2w, PDw. Almost no evidence of perfusion in first-pass images. Peripheral uptake in LGE images with hypointensity in the central part.

Conclusion These findings are consistent with the diagnosis of caseous necrosis. Caseous necrosis is a form of cell death in which the tissue maintains a cheese-like appearance. The dead tissue appears as a soft and white proteinaceous material. Frequently, caseous necrosis is encountered in the foci of tuberculosis infections. It can also be caused by syphilis and certain fungi.

Fig. 5.10 Still frame from cine sequence in short axis of left ventricle. Evidence of an ovoid mass close to the posterior leaflet of mitral valve. The mass has no infiltrative attitude. As an unexpected finding evidence of pericardial effusion of unknown origin and without any hemodynamic consequences

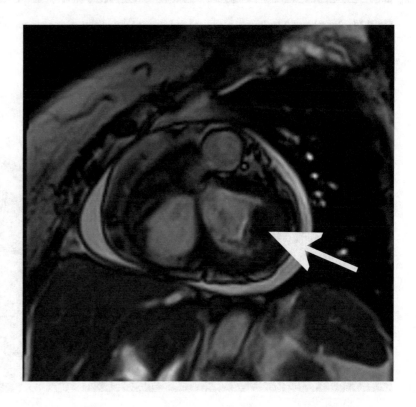

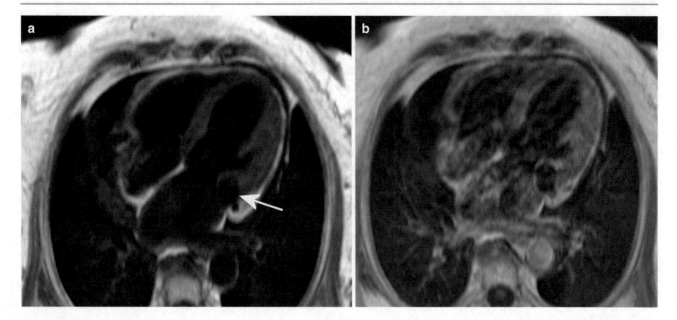

Fig. 5.11 Black blood T1w images before (**a**) and after (**b**) the administration of contrast agent. The ovoid mass shows a very low signal and no contrast enhancement

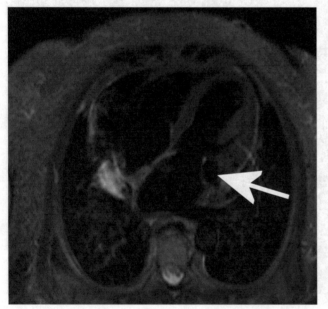

Fig. 5.12 Black blood T2w image with low intensity of the ovoid mass

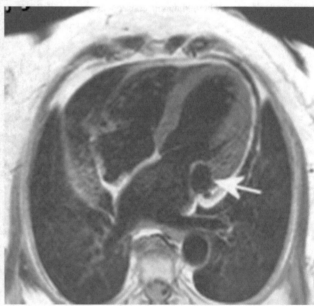

Fig. 5.13 Black blood PDw image with low intensity of the ovoid mass

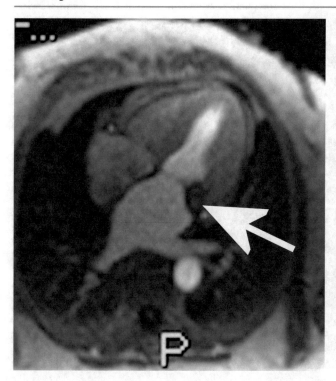

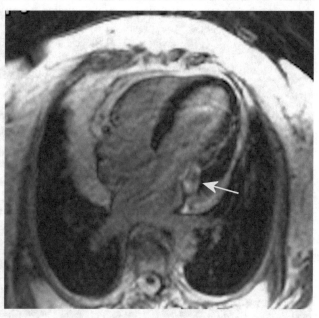

Fig. 5.15 LGE image with evidence of uptake of the c.a. in the peripheral part of the ovoid mass while the core shows low degree of enhancement

Fig. 5.14 GRE perfusion images. First-pass technique. Almost no perfusion is detectable within the ovoid mass

5.1.5 Fibroelastoma

Medical History Male, 83 y.o. Hypertension, previous prostatic cancer. Chronic atrial fibrillation. At Echocardiography evidence of small mass at the level of septal side of the left ventricle outflow tract.

CMR Flowchart Stack of cine images in short-axis view to evaluate biventricular volumes and function. Cine images in oblique view to show the presence, localization, and behav-

ior of the mass during the cardiac cycle. T1w, T2w, and LGE images to characterize the tissue of the mass.

Main CMR Findings Left-ventricle volume and global function normal. Presence of a round-shaped mass close to the interventricular septum at the level of the outflow tract (Movie 5.10 and Movie 5.11). The little mass (diameter 1 cm) shows good mobility and high signal intensity in T2w images, probably due to the presence of still blood within the mass itself. In LGE image the central core of the mass shows no uptake of contrast agent.

Conclusion Fibroelastoma.

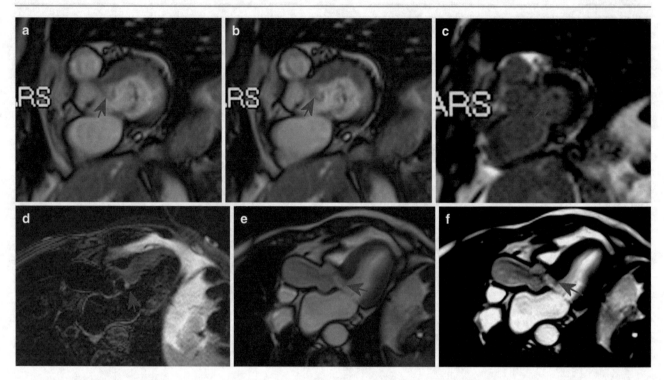

Fig. 5.16 (**a**) SSFP image in oblique view at the level of the outflow tract, early systolic frame; (**b**) SSFP image in the same oblique view, end-systolic frame; (**c**) LGE image: (**d**) T2w image in three-chamber view; (**e**) SSFP cine image in three-chamber view; (**f**) same image of (**e**) but after enhancing the contrast among structures. The arrows show the small (diameter 1 cm) and very mobile pathologic mass

5.1.6   Intra-atrial Schwannoma

Clinical History Female, 68 y.o. Three years earlier she underwent a surgical operation to remove a mass posteriorly to the mitral valve. The histological specimen resulted to be an intracardiac schwannoma.

One year later a further CMR study showed the mild left atrial wall thickening with no evidence of any mass.

One year later a new CMR evaluation showed a recidivism of the cardiac mass located at the level mitral valve with no evidence of fluid dynamic abnormalities.

CMR Flowchart SSFP cine images in vertical and horizontal planes. Stack of cine images to evaluate the biventricular global function. T1w, T2w, and T1w postcontrast and LGE images in oblique plane to evaluate the signal behavior of the intra-atrial mass.

Main CMR Findings Sizes and volumes of the ventricles are within normal range with the normal biventricular systolic function. Presence of a large intra-atrial mass close to the mitral valve plane, apparently not interfering with the mitral movement and the transvalvular flow (Movie 5.12 and Movie 5.13). The signal intensity appears to be dis-homogeneously hyperintense in all the sequences, while there is a central uptake in postcontrast T1w images.

Conclusion Presence of a recidivism of previously excised intra-atrial schwannoma.

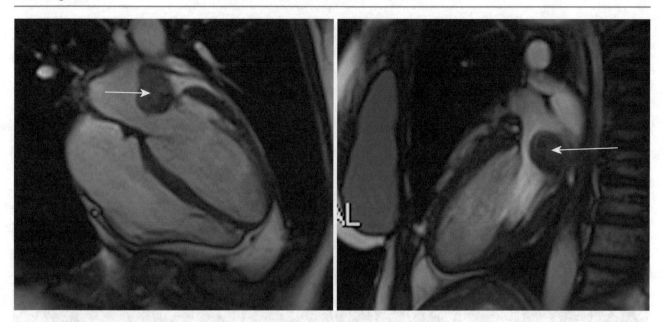

Fig. 5.17   SSFP cine images in horizontal long axis (left panel) and vertical long axis (right panel). Presence (arrows) of a round-shaped intra-atrial mass (27 × 25 × 27 mm (AP × LL × SI)) close to the mitral valve plane

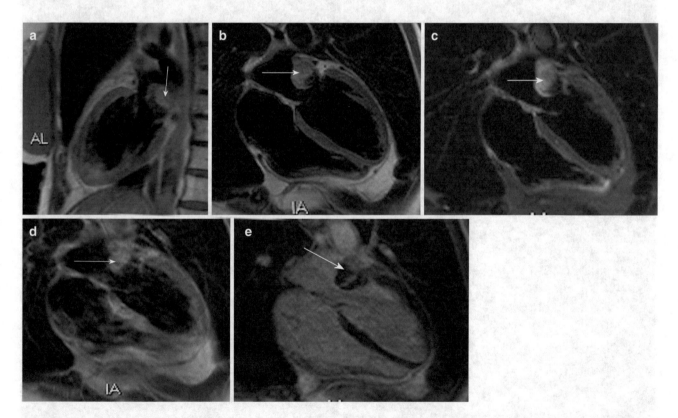

Fig. 5.18   Panel **a**: T1w image in vertical long axis; panel **b**: T1w image in horizontal long axis; panel **c**: T1w image fat saturation in horizontal long axis; **d**: T1w postcontrast image in horizontal long axis; **e**: postcontrast LGE image in horizontal long axis. Arrows show the intra-atrial mass

5.1.7   Rhabdomyoma

Medical History Female, 7 y.o. Sporadic extrasystolic activity. At transthoracic Echocardiography evidence of small hyperechogenic mass.

CMR Flowchart Stack of cine images in short-axis view to evaluate biventricular volumes and function and to identify the presence, extension, and hemodynamic consequences (if any) of the suspected mass. Black blood T1 and T2w images. LGE images.

Main CMR Findings Left-ventricle volume within limits with preserved global and regional function (EF 68%). Presence of a small, round-shaped mass at the level of the interventricular septum (Movie 5.14 and Movie 5.15). The mass has a behavior of the signal consistent with the native myocardium.

Conclusion Benign rhabdomyoma.

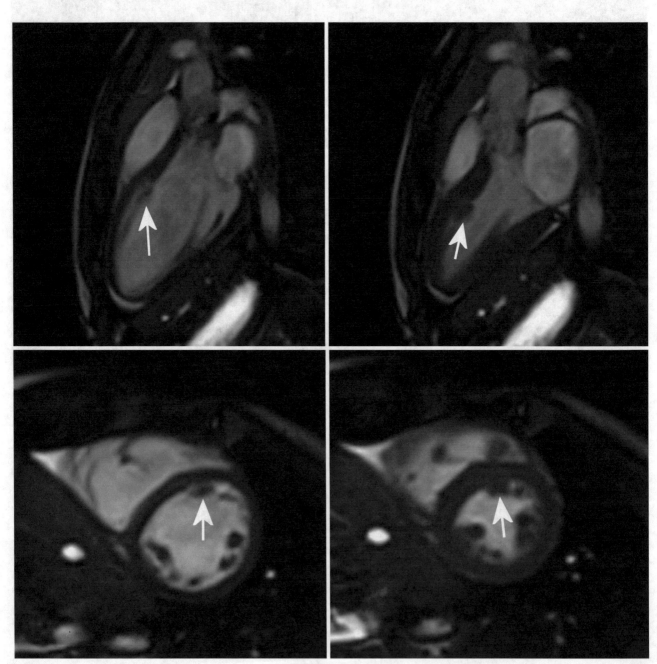

Fig. 5.19 SSFP cine images in vertical long axis (upper panels) and short axis of the heart (lower panels). The arrows show the intraventricular mass which is detectable either in end diastole (left panels) or in end systole (right panels)

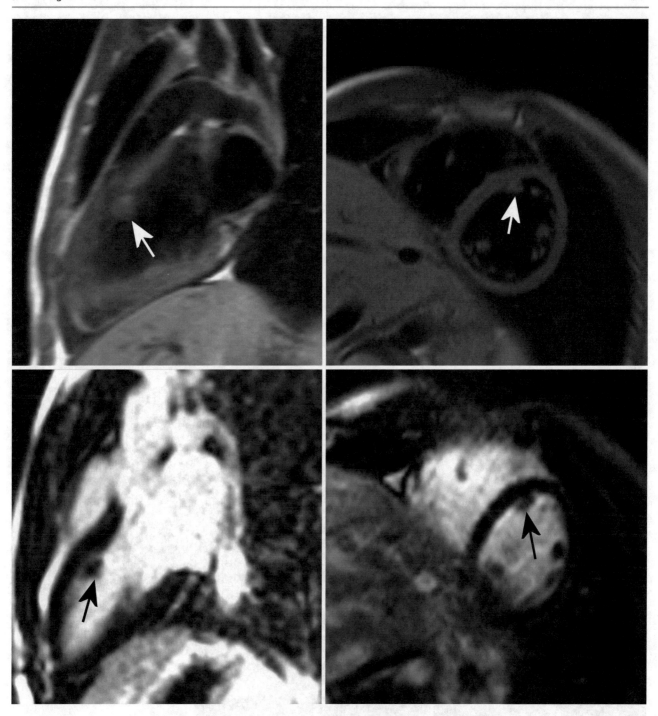

Fig. 5.20 T1w images (upper panels), T2w images (middle panels), and LGE images (lower panels). Vertical long axis (left panels) and short axis of the heart (right panels). The arrows show the round-shaped rhabdomyoma which has the same behavior of the myocardium in the different weighted images

5.1.8   Mediastinal Paraganglioma

Clinical History Twenty-five-year-old female patient with a history of gastrointestinal stromal tumor. After the surgical operation the patient was scanned by whole-body PET. Multiple areas of enhanced uptake of radiotracer: anterior abdominal wall, right cervical area, and mediastinal bilateral areas. Afterwards CT scan showed a mediastinal mass between the aorta and the pulmonary arteries.

The patient underwent also a genetic evaluation for the SDHC (succinate dehydrogenase complex subunit C) mutation which resulted positive. This gene has been considered responsible for the Carney-Stratakis syndrome. Urinary catecholamine test was also positive.

The next 123-I MIBG (IMetaiodobenzylguanidine) scintigraphy showed uptake in the accumulation in the thoracic region.

CMR Flowchart Stack of cine images in short-axis view to evaluate biventricular volumes and function and to identify the presence, extension, and hemodynamic consequences (if any) of the suspected mass. Cine images (SPSS) in oblique plane to evaluate the relationship with the surrounding structures and to drive the selection of scanning planes for the following images. Axial and T1-weighted and T2-weighted images to characterize the pathologic mass. Perfusion images to evaluate the first pass of a bolus of contrast agent (0.075 mmol/kg) through the mass itself. Adjunctive dose of contrast agent to reach the total dose of 0.2 mmol/kg. LGE images.

Main CMR Findings Presence of a large mass between the aortic arch and the pulmonary artery (Movie 5.16 and Movie 5.17). The signal intensity is isointense with respect to the myocardium in T1w while it is strongly hyperintense in T2w images.

The perfusion sequence shows a fast and intense first pass of the contrast agent through the mass, the latter being a consequence of the rich microvasculature of the mass itself (Movie 5.18).

Conclusion The tissue characteristics of the mass in the adopted sequences suggest a diagnosis of noninfiltrative paraganglioma of the mediastinum.

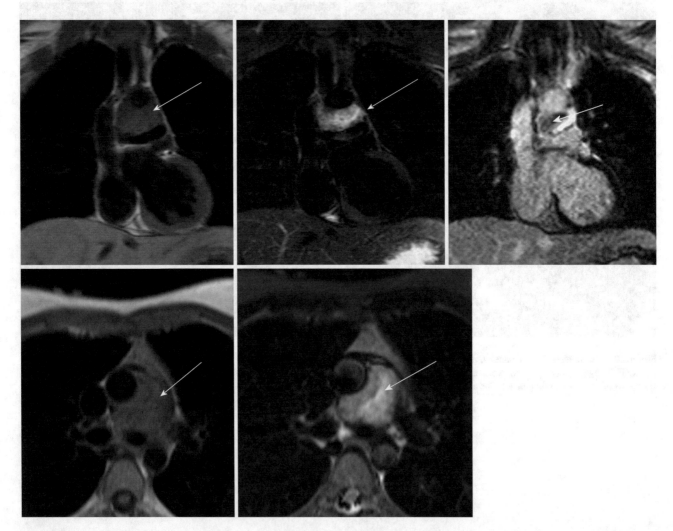

Fig. 5.21 Upper left panel and lower left panel: T1w images showing isointensity of the signal of the mass with respect to the myocardium. Upper middle panel and lower right panel: T2w images showing marked hyperintensity of the signal of the mass with respect to the myocardium. Upper right panel: LGE image showing a relatively low uptake of the contrast agent which is more pronounced in correspondence of the peripheral layer. Upper panels in coronal plane. Lower panels in axial plane

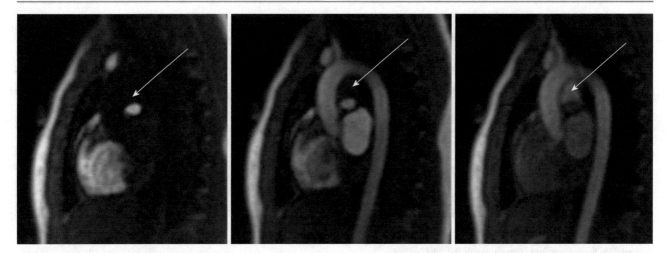

Fig. 5.22 Perfusion images. Three frames during the first pass of a bolus of contrast agent through the mediastinal mass. Left panel: image obtained with the contrast agent in the right ventricle and pulmonary arteries. Middle panel: image obtained during the arterial phase. Right panel: parenchymal contrastographic phase with pronounced level of signal intensity at the level of the pathologic mass

5.2 Malignant Tumors

5.2.1 Angiosarcoma

Medical History Male, 72 y.o. Palpitation. Dyspnea. Previous apparently successful surgical attempt to remove an angiosarcoma beside the right atrium. At recent echocardiographic examination suspect of recurrence of the tumoral disease.

CMR Flowchart Stack of cine images in short-axis view to evaluate biventricular volumes and function. Cine images in oblique view to obtain diagnostic images at the level of the right atrium. T1w and T2w images to better characterize the intra-atrial mass. First-pass images and postcontrast late enhancement to assess vascularization and tissue characteristics of the mass.

Main CMR Findings Left-ventricle volume and global function normal. In horizontal long axis (Movie 5.19) and in oblique view (Movie 5.20) evidence of an ovoid mass beside the right atrium. The atrial wall is not clearly detectable. The mass shows a inhomogeneous signal which is isointense in T1w and hyperintense in T2w images. During the first pass of a bolus of contrast agent only the peripheral layer shows increase of the signal while the central core shows little or no increase (Movie 5.21). The GRE-IR images collected late after the contrast agent injection show a clear uptake at the level of the peripheral layer with poor or no uptake within the central core.

Conclusion Recurrence of angiosarcoma which is apparently infiltrating the atrial wall.

Case provided by Dr. Sara Calamelli, Civil Hospital Mirano (VE), Italy.

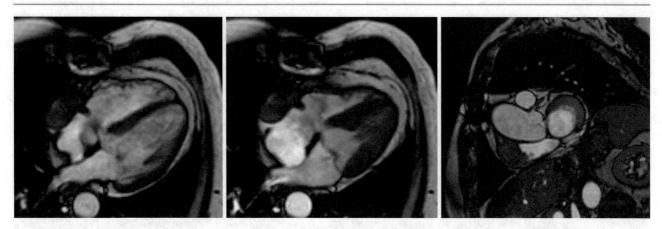

Fig. 5.23 SSFP cine images in horizontal long axis; left panel: end-diastolic frame, mid panel: end-systolic frame. In right panel an oblique view to complete the morphologic assessment of the tumoral mass

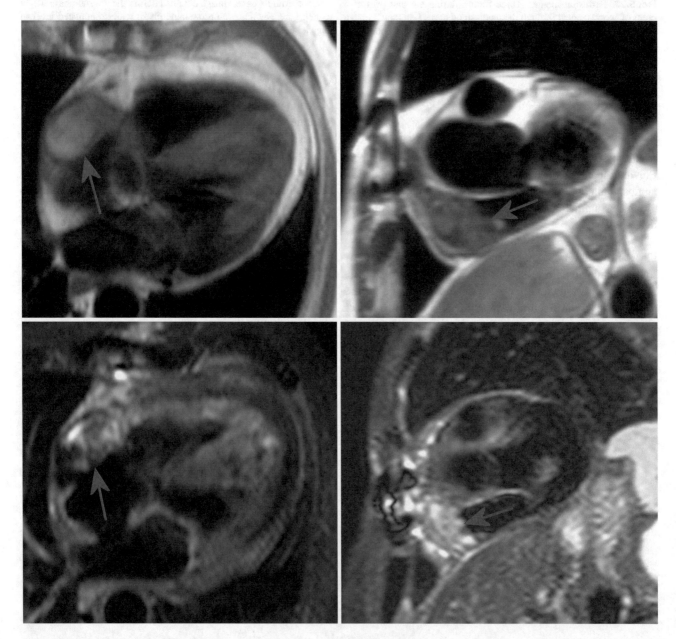

Fig. 5.24 Upper panels: T1w images in horizontal long-axis (left) and oblique (right) view (HR 95 b/min, TR 631 ms, TE 11 ms). Lower panels: T2w images in horizontal long-axis (left) and oblique (right) view (HR 94 b/min, TR 1894 ms, TE 100 ms). The arrows show the ovoid mass at the level of the right atrium

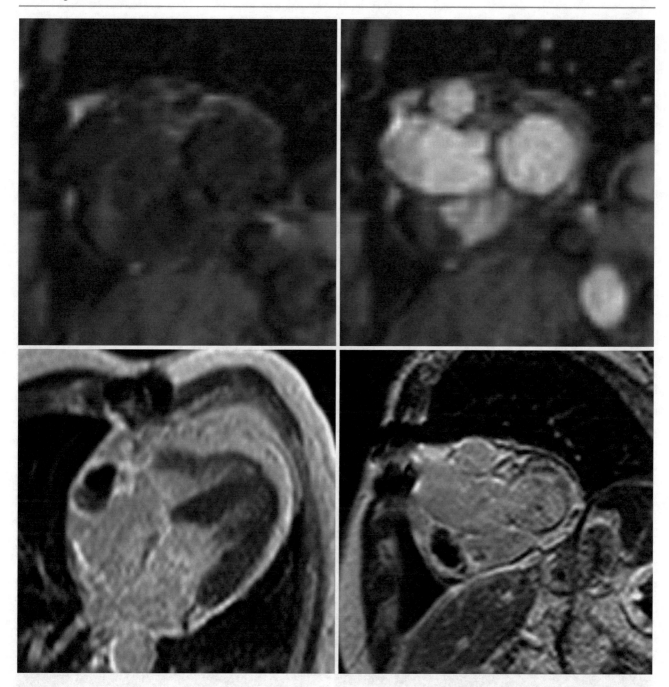

Fig. 5.25 Upper panels: first-pass perfusion images in oblique view across the tumoral mass. Images obtained before (left panel) and at peak increase of signal intensity. The tumoral mass does not show a significant increase of the signal but in the peripheral layer. Lower panels: LGE (GRE-IR) images obtained 10 min after the injection of con- trast agent. Left panel in horizontal long axis, right panel in oblique view. Evidence of little or no uptake of the contrast agent in the central core while a significant uptake is evident in the peripheral layer. These findings are presumably due to a reduced vascularization of the central core where extensive necrosis is also present

5.2.2 Recurrence of Angiosarcoma

Medical History Female, 13 y.o. Asymptomatic. Recent transthoracic echocardiographic control resulting to be normal.

CMR Flowchart Stack of cine images in short-axis view to evaluate biventricular volumes and function. Cine images in oblique view to obtain diagnostic images at the para-mediastinal mass. T1w and T2w images at the level of the pathologic mass. Contrast agent not administered due to previous severe allergic reaction.

Main CMR Findings Left-ventricle volume and global function normal. In cine images as well as in T1w and T2w images evidence of an ovoidal mass (33 × 33 × 26 mm; AP × LL × SI). In all kind of images dis-homogeneous signal (Movie 5.22).

Conclusion Recurrence of angiosarcoma.

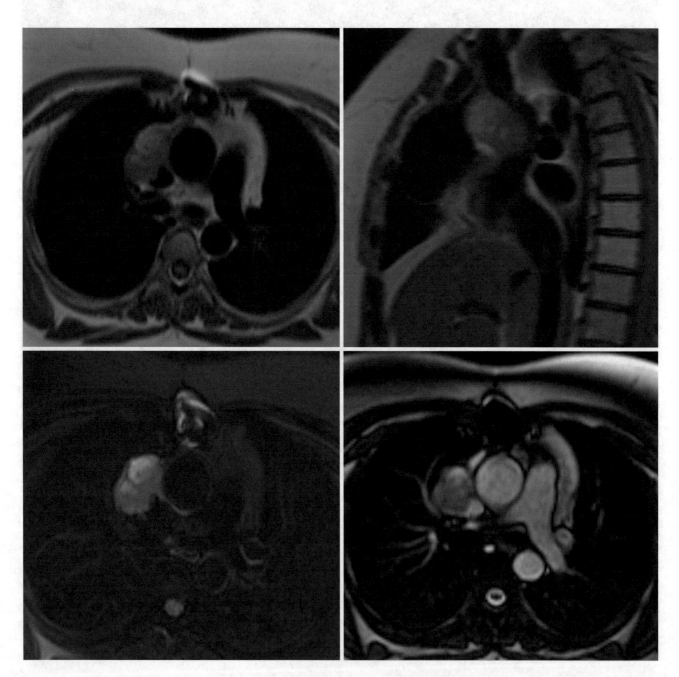

Fig. 5.26 Upper panels: T1w images in axial (left) and sagittal (right) view. Lower left panel: T2w image. Lower right panel: SSFP image at the level of the pulmonary bifurcation. In all images evidence of the tumoral mass which shows infiltrative nature at the level of the superior vena cava

5.2.3 Osteosarcoma

Medical History Male, 19 y.o. Palpitation, dyspnea.

CMR Flowchart Stack of cine images in short-axis view to evaluate biventricular volumes and function. Cine images in oblique view to obtain diagnostic images at the level of the tumoral mass and to evaluate the connection with the inferior vena cava. T1w and T2w to better define the tissue characteristics of the tumoral mass.

Main CMR Findings Left-ventricle volume and global function normal. Presence of a large inhomogeneous mass within the right side of the heart (Movie 5.23). The presence of the mass is detectable also at the level of the inferior vena cava which is partially occluded by the pathologic mass (Movie 5.24). A second, small mass is detectable at the level of the superior vena cava. The pathologic mass appears to be isointense in T1 and hyperintense in T2w. After contrast injection evidence of a marked uptake in T1 images. Evidence of infiltrative attitude of the pathologic masses.

Pleural and pericardial effusion.

Conclusion Osteosarcoma within the right side of the heart and obstacle to the venous return.

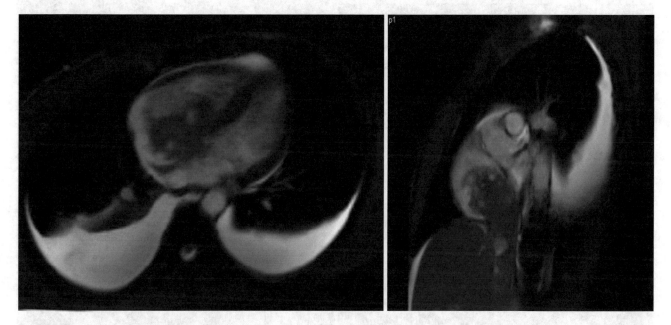

Fig. 5.27 SSFP cine images in horizontal long axis (left panel), and sagittal plane at the level of the inferior vena cava (right panel). Evidence of a large inhomogeneous mass occupying the right section of the heart and invading the inferior vena cava

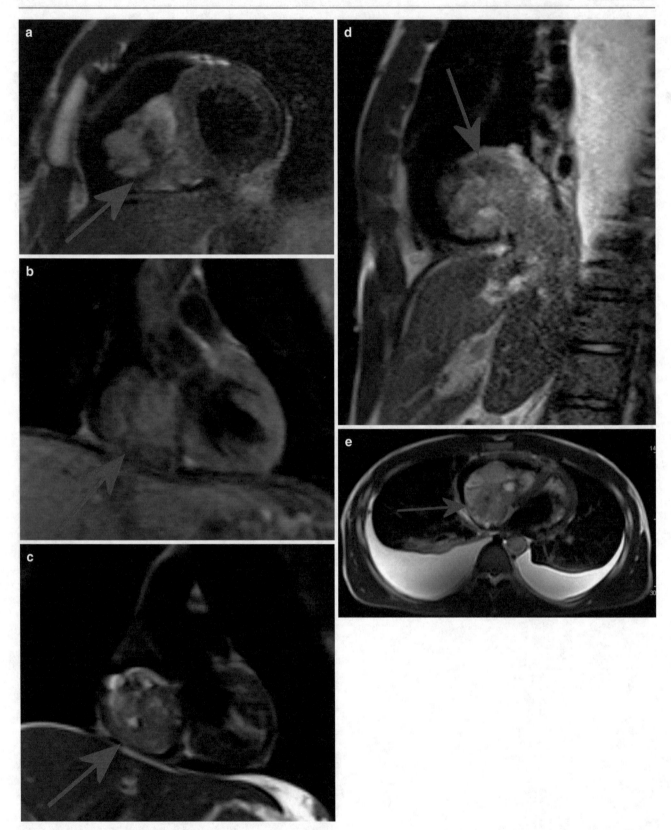

Fig. 5.28 Panels **a** and **d**: T2w image. Panel **b**: T1w image. Panels **c** and **e**: Proton density-weighted images. Evidence of a large inhomogeneous mass (arrows) which shows isointensity in T1w and PDw images while it is hyperintense in T2w images. Panel **e**: Evidence of large ammount of bilateral pleural effusion

5.2.4 Metastatic Mass (1)

Medical History Previous history of metastatic ovarian adenocarcinoma, diagnosed in 2011, operated (hysteroannessiectomy) and received chemotherapy. Under therapy with steroids because of systemic lupus erythematosus.

A previous echocardiogram showed severe systolic dysfunction of the left ventricle (LVEF = 24%), akinesia of the apex, and interventricular septum in the presence of hypokinesia of other segments. Currently asymptomatic.

CMR Flowchart Stack of cine images in short-axis view to evaluate biventricular volumes and function. Cine images in oblique view to evaluate the presence of metastatic structure and its relevance on cardiovascular dynamic. Images in Black Blood T1w and T2w to characterize the pathologic structure. Perfusion images (first pass) to assess the vascular component of the mass. Early postcontrast T1w images (FSE T1w) and late GRE-IR images (LGE).

Main CMR Findings Left-ventricle sizes and volumes and segmental wall thickness are normal. Global systolic function is severely depressed (LVEF = 33%) with diffuse hypo-

kinesia and akinesia of the apex and interventricular septum. Furthermore an intraventricular dys-synchrony is detectable.

Right-ventricle sizes and volumes are within the limits. Systolic function is within normal limits (RVEF = 57%).

In cine images a pathologic mass is detectable with 8 × 5 cm dimension (anteroposterior toward latero-lateral direction) (Movie 5.25 and Movie 5.26). The mass compresses the Superior Vena Cava and induces displacement of the right atrium.

In precontrast Black Blood T1 images the tumor is slightly hypo/isointense while it is hyperintense in T2w images. T1w postcontrast shows active uptake of the contrast media which can be interpreted as a tissue with relevant vascularization.

In the images acquired late after the administration of the contrast media (LGE) there is active uptake at the peripheral level while the core of the mass shows a quite reduced and inhomogeneous uptake.

Minimal pericardial effusion.

Conclusion The CMR findings are suggestive of a metastatic mass which is probably linked to the previous ovarian cancer.

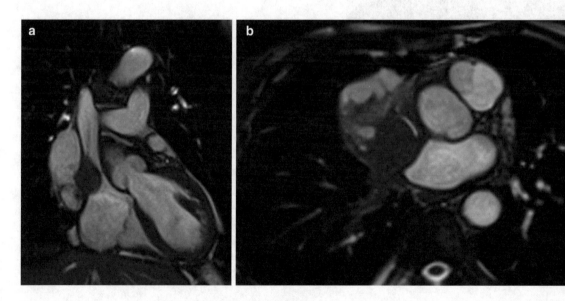

Fig. 5.29 (**a**) Still frame from a cine sequence (SSFP) in coronal view. Evidence of a tumoral mass at the level of the Superior Vena Cava whose diameter is strongly reduced due to the mass itself. (**b**) Still frame from a cine sequence acquired in axial plane. The tumoral mass is almost completely filling the right atrium, compressing the superior vena cava, and expanding outside the heart infiltrating the pulmonary hilum

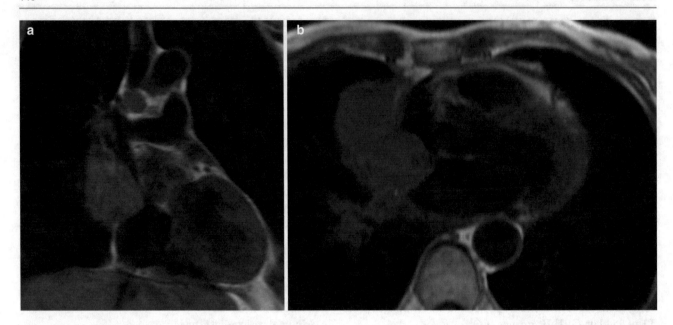

Fig. 5.30 Black Blood T1w images. The tumoral mass shows an isointense/slightly hyperintense signal with respect to the remote myocardium, (**a**) panel: coronal view, (**b**) panel: axial view

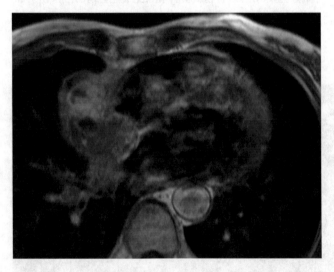

Fig. 5.31 Postcontrast T1w image. The tumoral mass shows an intense and inhomogeneous uptake of the contrast agent

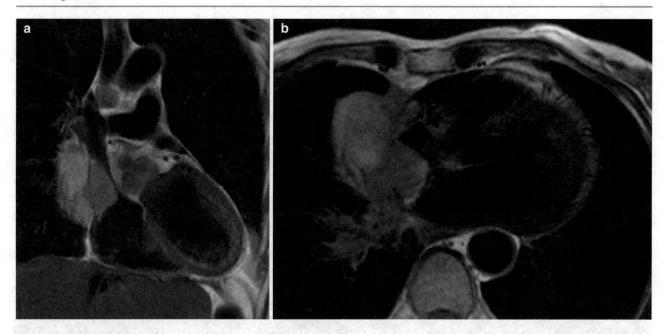

Fig. 5.32 Black Blood T2w images. Axial view. The tumoral mass shows an intense and inhomogeneous hyperintensity of the signal, (**a**) panel: coronal view, (**b**) panel: axial view

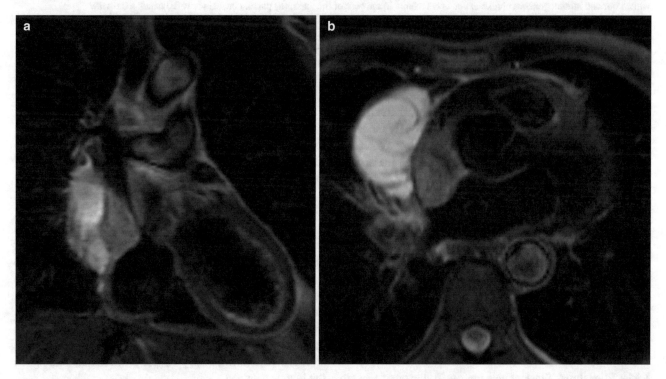

Fig. 5.33 T2w Black Blood triple inversion recovery images. The tumoral mass shows a relevant and quite inhomogeneous hyperintensity of the signal, presumably due to the presence of cystic component of the mass itself, (**a**) panel: coronal view, (**b**) panel: axial view

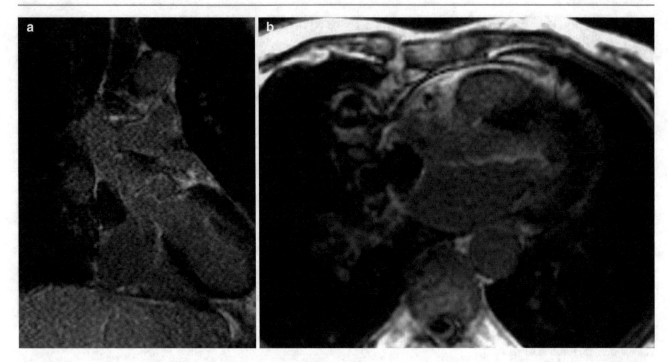

Fig. 5.34 Late postcontrast GRE IR (LGE) images. The tumoral mass shows a significant uptake of the contrast agent only on the peripheral rim while poor and inhomogeneous uptake of c.a. is detectable in the core of the mass, (**a**) panel: coronal view, (**b**) panel: axial view

5.2.5   Metastatic Mass (2)

Clinical History 54-year-old female patient with the history of a successfully operated 5 cm mass in the left leg with histological diagnosis of alveolar soft-part sarcoma. In 2003 radiotherapy because of multiple pulmonary metastasis. From 2004 till the day of examination numerous thermo-ablations, surgery procedures, and radiotherapy in lungs.

In 2018 therapy with pazopanib and anlotinib.

April 2018 at Echocardiography: LVEF = 63%, evidence of intramyocardial, expansive masses.

A CMR in 2018 showed multiple round-shaped intramyocardial neoformations at the level of right-ventricle outflow tract and lateral wall left ventricle. Total-body scintigraphy—negative.

October 2018 evidence of progression of disease at CT scan. Echocardiography: difficult acoustic window: LVEF = 50–55%.

CMR Flowchart Stack of cine images in short-axis view to evaluate biventricular volumes and function. Cine images in oblique view to evaluate the presence of metastatic structures and their relevance on cardiovascular dynamic. Black Blood T1w and T2w and LGE images on the masses. T1 mapping of myocardium as well as of the tumoral masses.

MR Report Normal sizes, volumes, and function of the left ventricle (LVEF = 67%). Impairment of regional function: hypokinesia of anteroseptal segment at basal and mid level.

Normal range of the sizes, volumes, and function of the right ventricle.

Presence of three myocardial lesions: a first one at the level of right-ventricle outflow tract but with no signs of obstruction (Movie 5.27), a second mass at the level of the left ventricle apex, and a third mass at the level of the left-ventricle lateral wall with evidence of myocardial infiltration.

Myocardial T1 values are slightly elevated, possibly due to the fibrosis related to chemotherapy.

It is also confirmed the presence of metastatic findings in the lung and spleen.

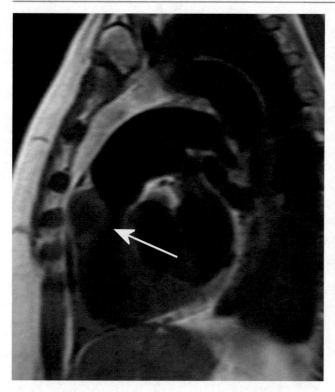

Fig. 5.35 Proton density image at the level of the right ventricular outflow tract. Parasagittal plane. Evidence of the metastatic mass at the level of the outflow tract (arrow)

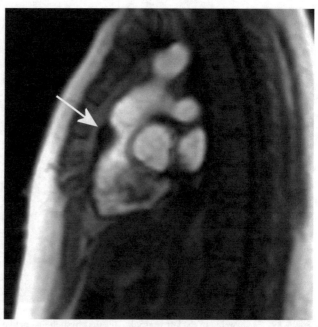

Fig. 5.37 Perfusion image at the level of the right ventricular outflow tract. Parasagittal plane. Evidence of the metastatic mass at the level of the outflow tract (arrow). The image shows a hyper-vascularized peripheral layer of the mass while the central core is necrotic and hypo-vascularized (darker)

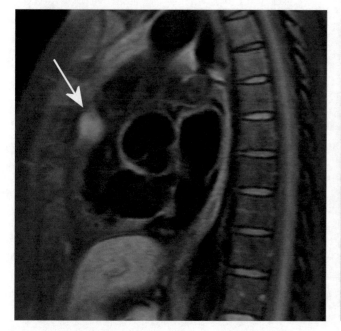

Fig. 5.36 T2-weighted image at the level of the right ventricular outflow tract. Parasagittal plane. Evidence of the metastatic mass at the level of the outflow tract (arrow)

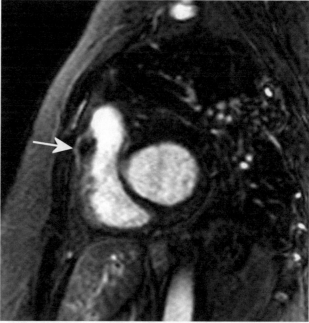

Fig. 5.38 LGE image of the mass showing a slight hyper-enhanced peripheral layer while the central core is hypo-enhanced due to the prevalence of necrotic tissue

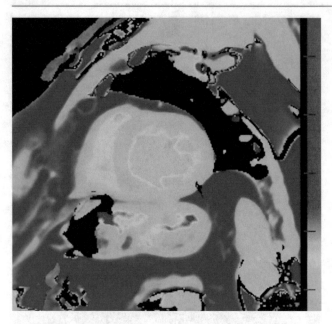

Fig. 5.39 T1 mapping of the left ventricle. Results are such that native T1 value is 1013 ms while ECV resulted to be 29%

5.3   Intracardiac Thrombosis

5.3.1   Left-Ventricle Apical Thrombosis

Medical History Male, 50 y.o. Acute myocardial infarction 2 months before the CMR study. Coronary bypass 1 month before the CMR study.

CMR Flowchart Cine images in vertical and horizontal long axis. Stack of cine images in short-axis view to evaluate biventricular volumes and function. T2w images in short and long axes. LGE images acquired early (3 min) (long TI) and late (10 min) (optimized TI) after the administration of c.a. (0.2 mmol/kg).

Main CMR Findings Regional and global impairment of LV function (EF 37%). Extended apical necrosis partially transmural (>75% of transmurality). Presence of apical thrombosis (18 × 11 × 9 mm, SI × AP × LL) (Movie 5.28 and Movie 5.29) which shows high-intensity signal in T2w image.

Conclusion Recent myocardial infarction complicated by apical thrombosis. The high intensity of the signal in T2w image depends on the recent nature of the thrombotic process.

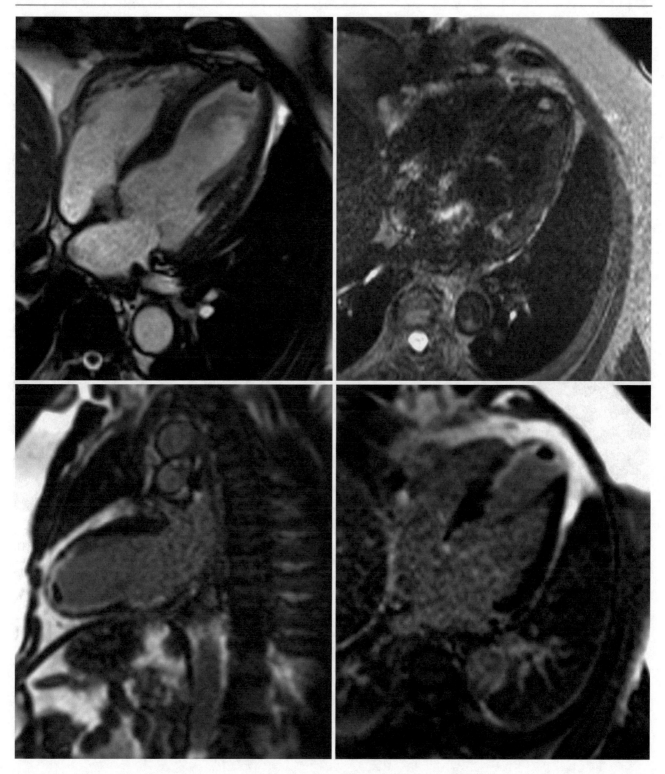

Fig. 5.40 Left upper panel. Still frame from a SSFP cine sequence. Presence of a thrombotic mass at the level of the apex. Right upper panel: T2w image from the same patient. Despite the low quality of the image the thrombus is detectable at the level of the apex as a hyperintense mass. This probably due to the recent formation of the thrombus. In the lower panels LGE images in vertical (left) and horizontal (right panel) long axis of the heart. Presence of the thrombus at the level of the apex surrounded by a large necrotic scar involving all the apical and inferior segments

5.3.2 Previous AMI, Large Apical Thrombus

Medical Hystory Male, 67 y.o.

Previous acute myocardial infarction. Late arrival to the emergency room (after 1 week from the onset of symptoms). Dyspnea.

At angiography, occlusion of anterior descending artery and II diagonal branch.

CMR Flowchart SSFP cine images in horizontal and vertical long axis. Stack of cine images in short-axis view to eval-uate biventricular volumes and function. Postcontrast LGE images to evaluate the presence and location of postischemic scar and to detect the presence of intraventricular thrombotic mass.

Main CMR Findings Severe depression of LV function (EF 29%) with large anterior-apical scar and presence of a large apical thrombotic mass (Movie 5.30).

Conclusion Previous anterior myocardial infarction with intraventricular thrombus. Severe reduction of LV function.

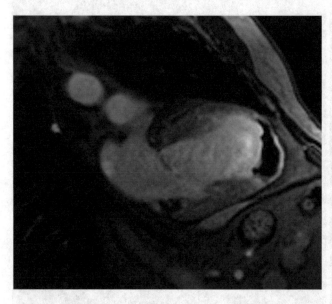

Fig. 5.41 Postcontrast GRE-IR images. Early acquisition (3 min) after c.a. (0.18 mmol/kg) injection. Maintaining the time of inversion (TI) relatively high (400 ms). TR 1800 ms

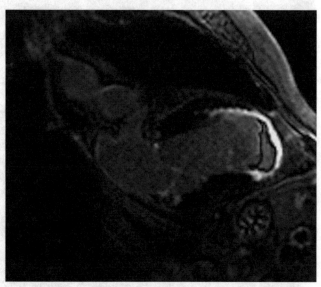

Fig. 5.42 Postcontrast GRE-IR images. Late acquisition (10 min) after c.a. (0.18 mmol/kg) injection. Maintaining the time of inversion (TI) such to null the signal from normal myocardium (270 ms). TR 1800 ms. With respect to the previous image there is a diffuse enhancement of the thrombotic stratification

Bibliography

1. Lombardi M, Plein S, Petersen S, Bucciarelli-Ducci C, Valsangiacoo Buechel M, Basso C, Ferrari V, editors. The EACVI textbook of cardiovascular magnetic resonance. Oxford: Oxford University Press; 2018.
2. Robbins SL, Kumar V. Robbins and Cotran: pathologic basis of disease. 8th ed. Philadelphia: Saunders; 2010. p. 16.
3. Pazos-López P, Pozo E, Siqueira ME, García-Lunar I, Cham M, Jacobi A, Macaluso F, Fuster V, Narula J, Sanz J. Value of CMR for the differential diagnosis of cardiac masses. JACC Cardiovasc Imaging. 2014;7(9):896–905.
4. Takashima Y, Kamitani T, Kawanami S, Nagao M, Yonezawa M, Yamasaki Y, Baba S, Yabuuchi H, Hida T, Kohashi K, Nakamura K, Sonoda H, Oda Y, Honda H. Mediastinal paraganglioma. Jpn J Radiol. 2015;33(7):433–6.
5. Basso C, Buser PT, Rizzo S, Lombardi M, Thiene G. Masses and tumors. In: Lombardi M, Plein S, Petersen S, Bucciarelli-Ducci C, Valsangiacoo Buechel M, Basso C, Ferrari V, editors. The EACVI textbook of cardiovascular magnetic resonance. Oxford: Oxford University Press; 2018.
6. Hoffmann U, Globits S, Schima W, Loewe C, Puig S, Oberhuber G, Frank H. Usefulness of magnetic resonance imaging of cardiac and paracardiac masses. Am J Cardiol. 2003;92(7):890–5.
7. Saba SG, Bandettini PW, Shanbhag SM, Spottiswoode BS, Kellman P, Arai AE. Characterization of cardiac masses with T1 mapping. J Cardiovasc Magn Reson. 2015;17(Suppl 1):Q32.

Pericardial Diseases

6.1 Acute Pericarditis

Medical History Male, 58 y.o. Dyslipidemia, hypercholesterolemia, ex-smoker. Five months earlier, he was admitted to the emergency room because of typical chest pain. ECG: diffuse ST-segment abnormalities, increased, CRP and HS-troponin. Despite optimized medical therapy a second episode of typical chest pain 2 weeks before the current CMR exam.

CMR Flowchart Stack of cine images in short-axis view to evaluate biventricular volumes and function. T2w images in short- and long-axis views. LGE images in short- and long-axis views after the injection of a bolus of contrast agent (0.2 mmol/kg).

Main CMR Findings Normal biventricular regional and global function. Normal thickness of left-ventricle walls. Thickening of pericardial layers which appear hyperintense in T2w images and show diffuse uptake of c.a. in LGE images. Spotty subepicardial uptake of c.a. No pericardial effusion (Movie 6.1).

Conclusion Pericarditis with minimum subepicardial involvement and without pericardial effusion.

Electronic Supplementary Material The online version of this chapter (https://doi.org/10.1007/978-3-030-41830-4_6) contains supplementary material, which is available to authorized users.

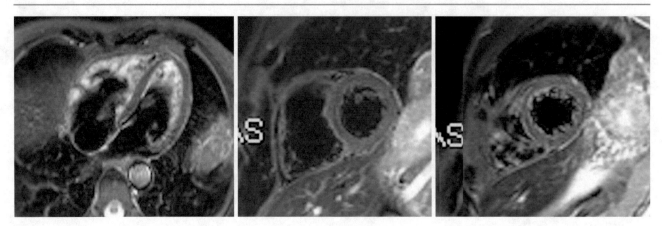

Fig. 6.1 T2w images in horizontal long axis (left panel) and short axis of the left ventricle (middle and right panels) showing diffuse hyperintensity at the level of the pericardium due to the presence of tissue edema

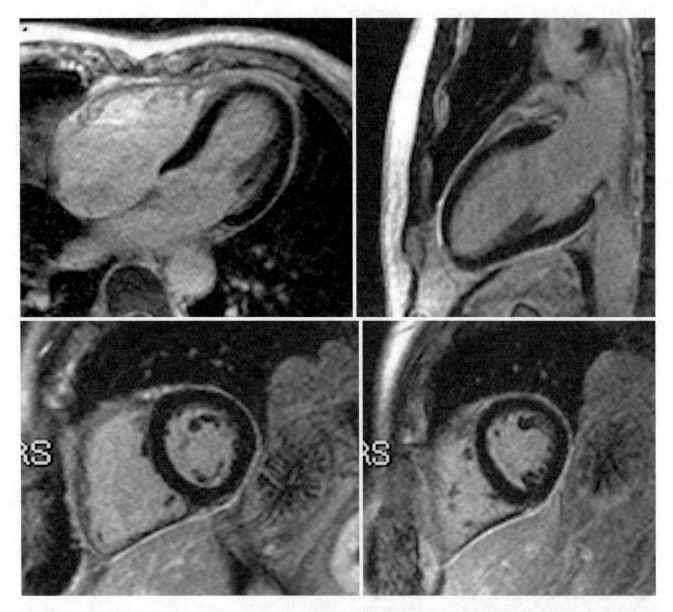

Fig. 6.2 LGE images obtained 10 min after the e.v. injection of paramagnetic c.a. A diffuse uptake of c.a. is evident in all the projections. Upper left panel: horizontal long axis. Upper right panel: vertical long axis. Lower panels: two parallel images of the heart in short axis

6.2   Acute Pericarditis with Pericardial Effusion

Medical History   Female, 40 y.o. Acute chest pain and pathologic biohumoral parameters.

CMR Flowchart   Stack of cine images in short-axis view to evaluate biventricular volumes and function. T2w images in short and long axis view to detect the presence of edema. LGE images in short and long axis view to detect myocardial fibrosis.

Main CMR Findings   Normal biventricular volumes and function. Abnormal increase of signal at the level of pericardium in T2w images. Shadow uptake of contrast agent at the level of inferolateral distal wall. Diffuse pericardial effusion with no hemodynamic meaning (Movie 6.2 and Movie 6.3).

Conclusion   Acute pericarditis with pericardial effusion.

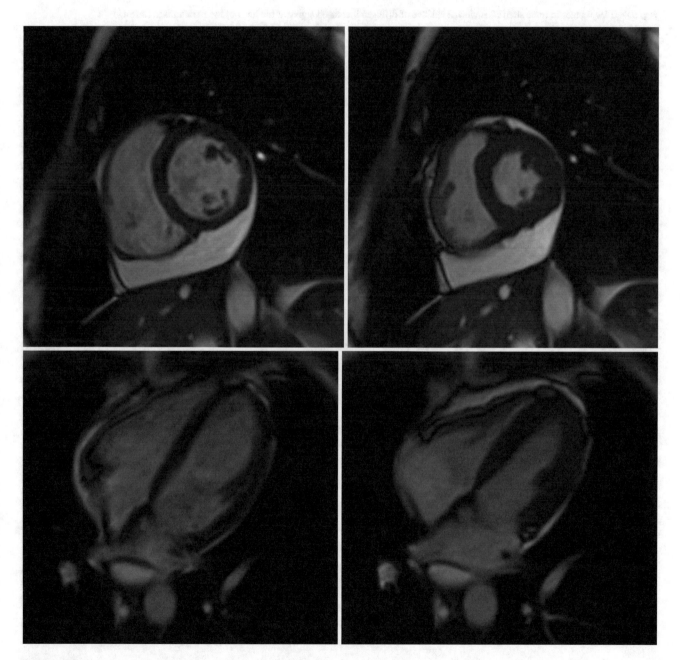

Fig. 6.3 SSFP cine images in short-axis view (upper panels) and in horizontal long-axis view (lower panels). Evidence of pericardial effusion which is visible either in diastole (left panels) or in systole (right panels)

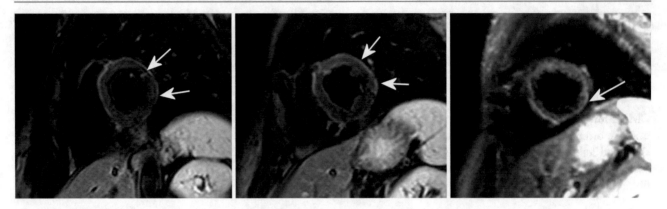

Fig. 6.4 T2w images in three short-axis view. Evidence of diffused increased signal at the level of the pericardium (arrows)

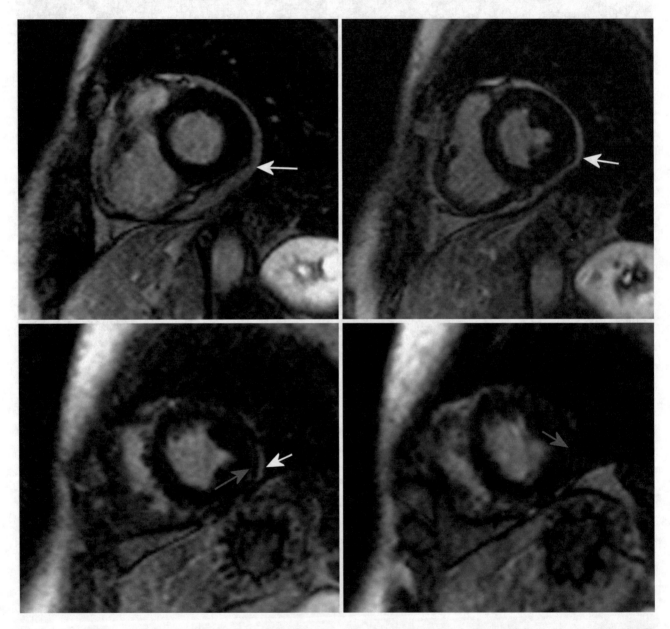

Fig. 6.5 LGE images. Four parallel short-axis views of the heart. The white arrows show diffuse pericardial effusion. The red arrows show a shadowed pericardial uptake of contrast agent in correspondence of the inferolateral segment

6.3   Chronic Pericarditis with Pericardial Effusion

Medical History   Male, 14 y.o. Idiopathic pericardial effusion.

CMR Flowchart   Stack of cine images in short-axis view to evaluate biventricular volumes and function. Cine images in vertical, horizontal and three chambers view Black Blood T2w images in short and long axis view to detect/exclude the presence of edema. LGE images in short axis view and vertical and long axis view.

Main CMR Findings   Left-ventricle volume and global function normal. Massive pericardial effusion. Thickening of pericardial visceral layer (Movie 6.4, Movie 6.5, Movie 6.6 and Movie 6.7).

Conclusion   Massive pericardial effusion in chronic pericarditis.

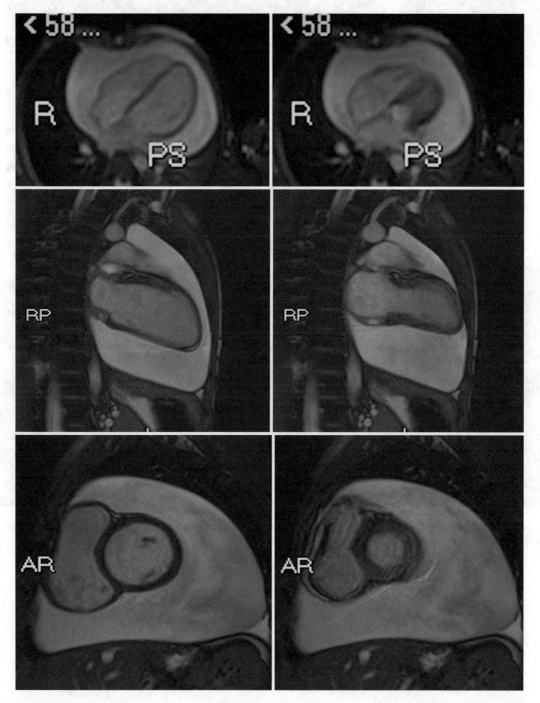

Fig. 6.6   Real-time free-breathing cine images obtained SSFP in horizontal long-axis view (upper panels), SSFP cine images in vertical long-axis (middle panels) and short-axis (lower panels) views. Left panels: images obtained at end diastole. Right panels: images obtained at end systole. Evidence of massive pericardial effusion

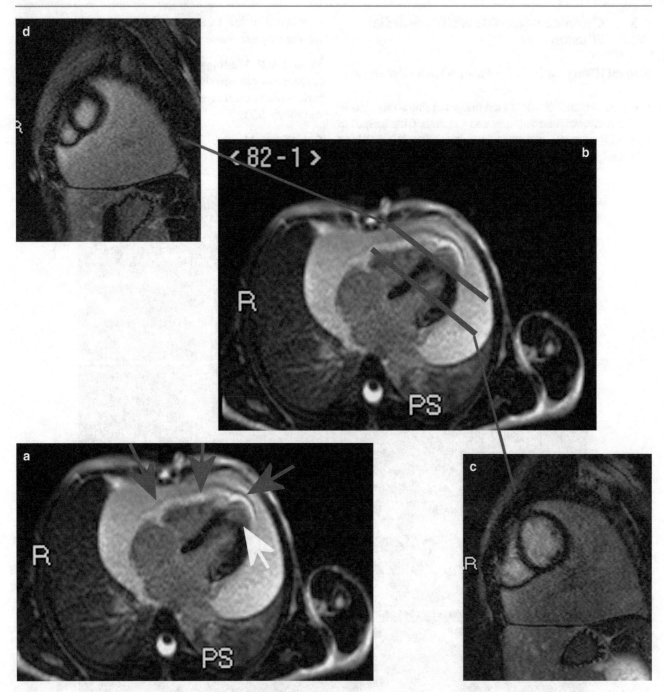

Fig. 6.7 Postcontrast LGE images. (**a**) Horizontal long axis. The red arrows show a diffuse thickened pericardium. The white arrow shows a suspected apical uptake of contrast agent. However obtaining orthogo- nal planes as shown in panel **b** there is no evidence of uptake (panels **c** and **d**)

6.4 Constrictive Pericarditis

Medical History Male, 63 y.o. Previous pancreatitis, nephrotic syndrome. Previous acute pericarditis. Pronounced swelling of body tissues (anasarca).

CMR Flowchart Stack of cine images in short-axis view to evaluate biventricular volumes and function. Cine images in multiple long-axis views (horizontal, vertical, three chambers view, etc). Phase-contrast images at the level of the tricuspid and mitral valve either during deep inspiration and expiration to assess the ventricular interdependency. Black Blood PDw, T1w, T2w, and LGE images to characterize the pericardium and the pericardial effusion.

Main CMR Findings Reduced biventricular volumes with preserved global function. Paradoxical movement of the interventricular septum. Increased interdependency of ventricles. Diffuse increased thickness of the pericardium (Movie 6.8, Movie 6.9 and Movie 6.10).

Conclusion Constrictive pericarditis.

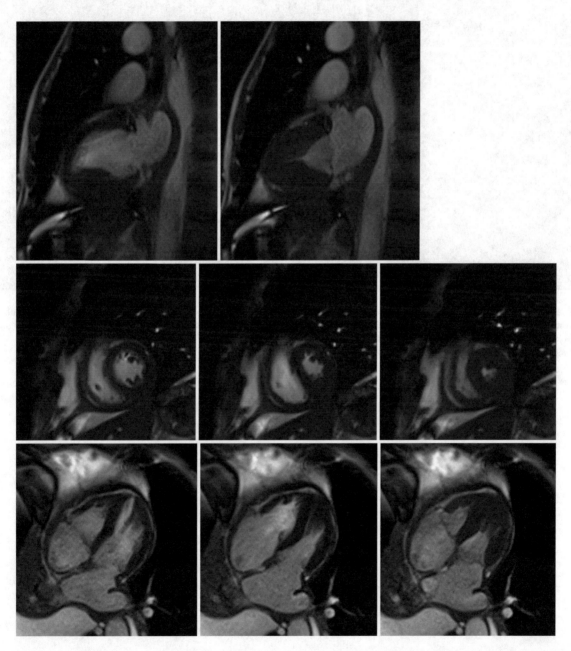

Fig. 6.8 SSFP images in vertical long axis (upper panels). Evidence of reduced volumes and preserved global function. In middle panels images in short-axis view of the heart. Left panel: end-diastolic frame. Middle panel in early diastolic phase with evidence of D-shaped movement. Middle right panel: end-systolic frame. In lower panels (horizontal long-axis view): left panel: end-diastolic frame, middle panel in early diastolic phase with evidence of paradoxical movement of the interventricular septum. Middle right panel: end-systolic frame

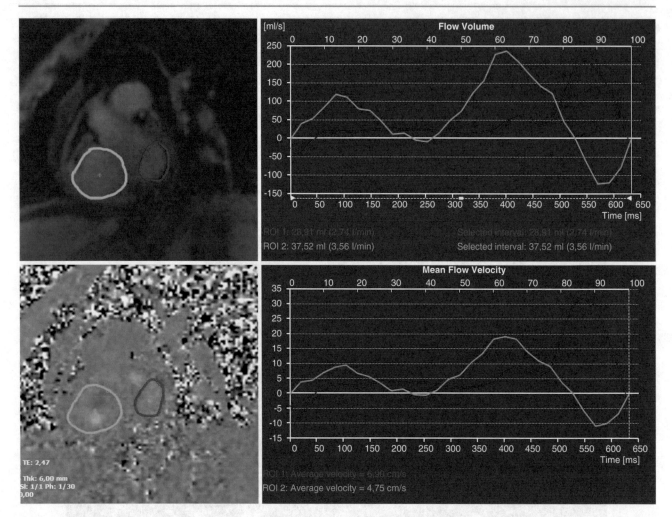

Fig. 6.9 Phase-contrast images positioned at the level of the valvular plane to measure simultaneously the flow through the mitral and the tricuspid valve. Upper left panel: magnitude image. Left lower panel: flow image. Right panels: diagram of the transvalvular flow (red through the mitral valve, green through the tricuspid valve) obtained in deep inspiration (upper right panel) and expiration (lower right panel). Evidence of interdependency of ventricle filling

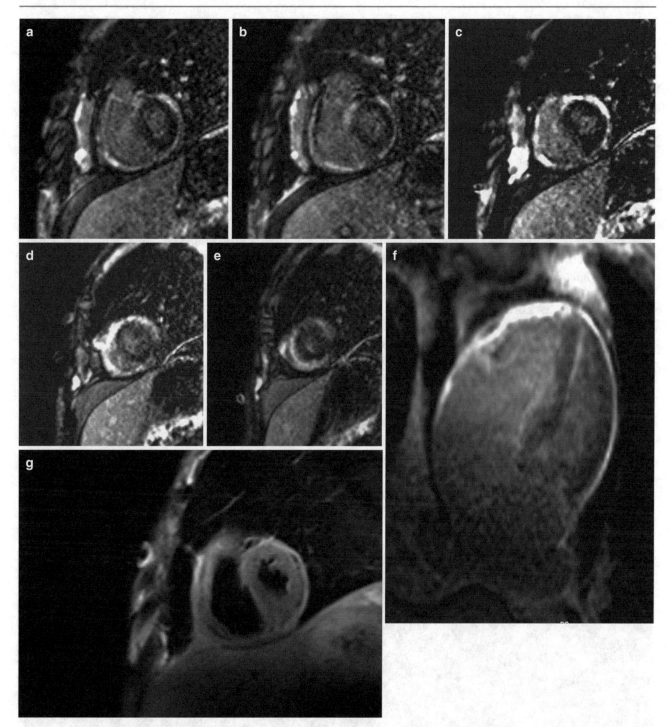

Fig. 6.10 Panels (**a–e**): LGE images in five parallel short-axis view of the heart. Panel **f**: LGE image in horizontal long-axis view. Panel **g**: PDw image. Evidence of diffuse severely increased thickness of the pericardium

6.5 Constrictive Pericarditis in Sarcoidosis

Clinical History Female, 54-year-old patient, with the history of cutaneous Sarcoidosis and cardiac involvement. Development of constrictive pericarditis.

Transthoracic Echocardiography showed normal-sized left ventricle with slightly impaired systolic function (LVEF = 49%). Presence of wall motion abnormalities: hypokinesia of the inferior and lateral wall (basal-mid segments). Calcification of the posterior leaflet of the mitral valve with no regurgitation. Severe dilatation of the left atrium. Right-ventricle free wall showed diffuse hypokinesia. No severe tricuspid regurgitation. Thickening and calcification of the pericardial layers in correspondence of the right-ventricle free wall and the inferolateral wall of the left ventricle.

CMR Flowchart Stack of cine images in short-axis view to evaluate biventricular function. Black blood T1w and T2w images. Postcontrast T1w images or perfusion images at the level of nodular/pericardial pathologic findings to indirectly evaluate the level of vascularity. Postcontrast late-enhancement GR E-IR images.

Main CMR Findings Sizes and volumes of the left ventricle are at the lower normal limits in the presence of mild reduction in systolic function (LVEF = 46%) because of global hypokinesia.

Sizes and volumes of the right ventricle are normal with a normal global systolic function (LVEF = 47%). Reduced expandability of RV anterior free wall (Movie 6.11 and Movie 6.12).

Biatrial dilatation.

In black blood T1- and T2-weighted images presence of nodular formations at epicardial/pericardial level which show a consistent low signal intensity in all kind of images. This behaviour is compatible with their calcific nature.

After the administration of the contrast media no presence of fibrosis. No enhancement of the nodular structure.

The thickening of the pericardium is remarkable (maximum thickness in correspondence of the inferior wall: 5.5 mm, in correspondence of the anterior wall 15 mm).

Regarding the analysis of the trans-mitral and trans-tricuspid flows there is a clear evidence of the significant interdependency between the two transvalvular flows:

– In inspiration trans-mitral flow 2.42 l/min, trans-tricuspid flow 2.07 l/min
– In expiration trans-mitral flow 2.24 l/min, trans-tricuspid flow 1.41 l/min

Remarkable dilatation of the inferior vena cava.

Conclusion Based on the cutaneous biopsy positive for Sarcoidosis and the nodular findings at the level of the heart the final diagnosis resulted in cardiac Sarcoidosis with evidence of constrictive pericarditis. Patient underwent positron-emission tomography and right-heart catheterization which confirmed the diagnostic suspect.

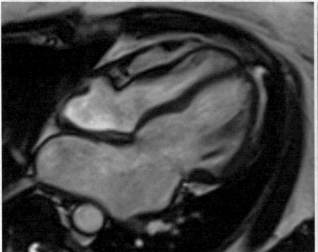
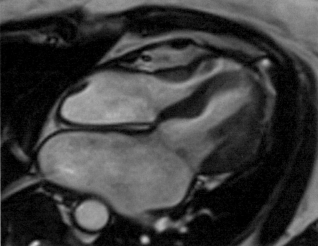

Fig. 6.11 Cine images (SSFP). Horizontal long axis. Evidence of thickened pericardium and tube-shape right ventricle. Left panel: end-diastolic frame. Right panel: end-systolic frame

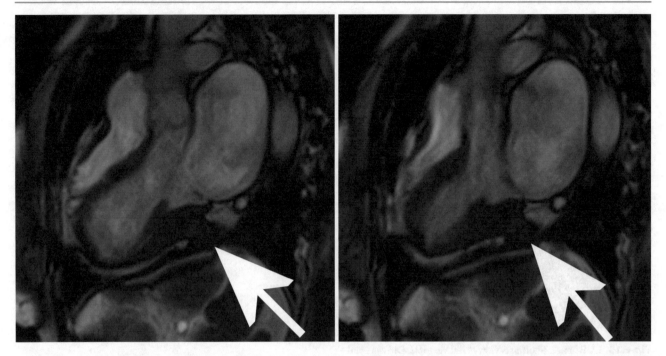

Fig. 6.12 Cine images (SSFP). Vertical long axis. Evidence of thickened pericardium and presence of epicardial/pericardial nodule (arrow). Left panel: end-diastolic frame. Right panel: end-systolic frame

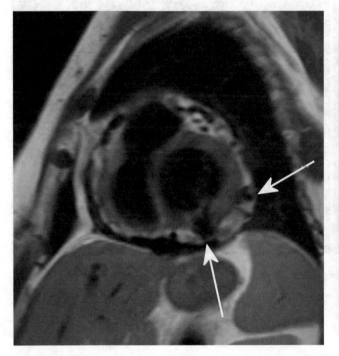

Fig. 6.13 T1w image. Short-axis view of the left ventricle. The arrows show the epicardial/pericardial nodules whose signal intensity is very low

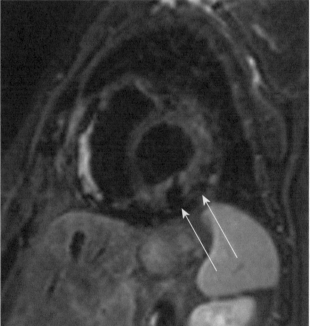

Fig. 6.14 T2w image. Short-axis view of the left ventricle. The arrows show the epicardial/pericardial nodules which show a very low signal intensity

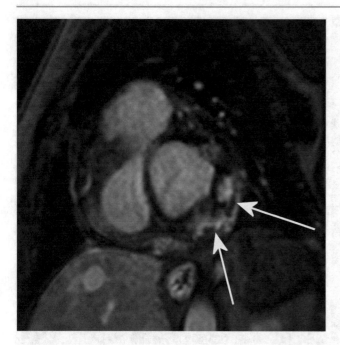

Fig. 6.15 LGE image. Short-axis view of left ventricle. Diffuse uptake around the hypointense nodules (arrows)

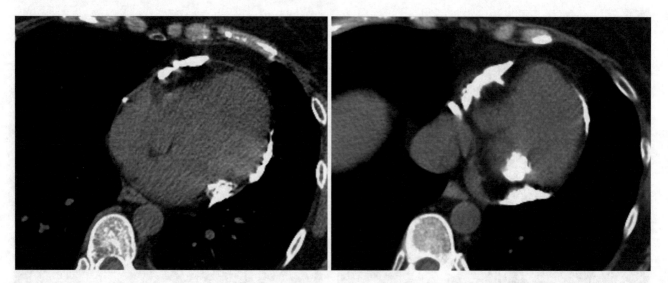

Fig. 6.16 CT images. Presence of diffuse calcification at the level of the pericardium (left panel) and at the level of the nodules (right panel)

6.6 Pericardial Diverticulum

Medical History Female, 73 y.o. Asymptomatic. Abnormal right-heart silhouette at chest X-Ray performed because of persistent cough. The latter successfully treated with antibiotic therapy.

CMR Flowchart Stack of GRE T1 images in axial planes to identify the presence and location of abnormal findings on a morphologic base. Stack of cine images in short-axis view to evaluate biventricular volumes and function. Cine SSFP, T1w, T2w, T2 fat saturation, T1 postcontrast and LGE images in orthogonal planes to characterize the abnormal finding.

Main CMR Findings Presence of a fluid-filled mass beside the ascending aorta (Movie 6.13). The mass is isointense in T1w images and hyperintense in T2w images. There is no suppression in fat saturation, and no uptake of contrast agent. There is evidence of coexistence of pericardial effusion (Movie 6.14).

Conclusion The signal characteristics and the coexistence of pericardial effusion as well as the location are consistent with the diagnosis of pericardial diverticulum.

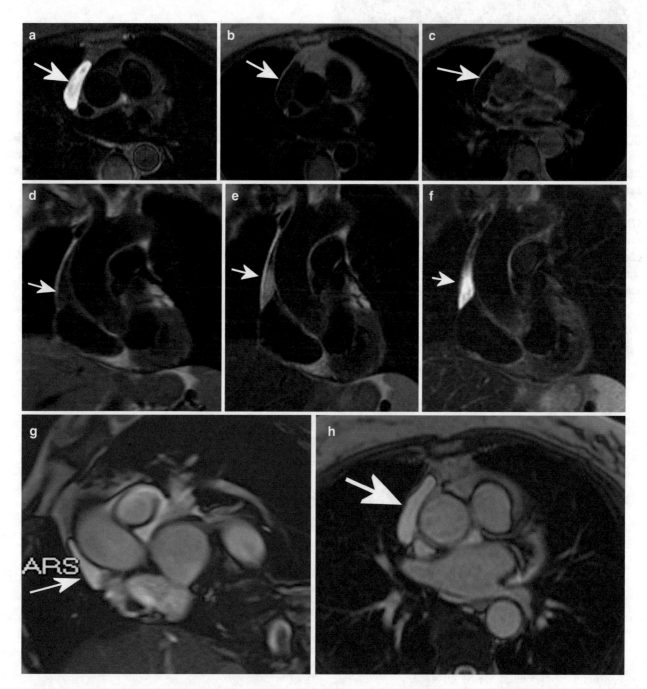

Fig. 6.17 Images of the abnormal mass obtained with different weighting: (**a**) T2w fat saturation image in axial plane; (**b**) same plane in T1w image; (**c**) same plane in T1w image 3 min after the administration of contrast; (**d**) T1w image in coronal plane; (**e**) T2w image in coronal plane; (**f**) T2w fat saturation image in coronal plane; (**g**) SSFP image in an oblique plane; (**h**) Gradient Echo T1w image in axial plane

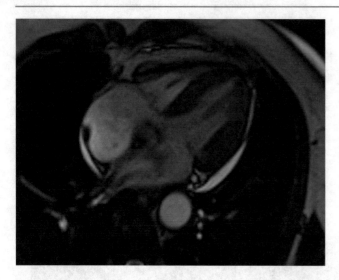

Fig. 6.18 SSFP cine sequence. Systolic frame. Evidence of pericardial fluid

6.7   Pericardial Agenesis

Medical History Male, 10 y.o. Asymptomatic. Abnormal cardiac silhouette at chest X-Ray.

CMR Flowchart Stack of cine images in short-axis view to evaluate biventricular volumes and function. Stack of SSFP cine images in horizontal long axis. Proton density images in short and horizontal long axis. LGE images in short and horizontal long axis.

Main CMR Findings Left-ventricle volume and global function normal. Shift of the mediastinal mass toward left. Presence of indentation on the right-ventricle free wall (Movie 6.15). No evidence of the pericardial layer either in cine images or in PD images. No uptake of c.a. in LGE images.

Conclusion Pericardial agenesis.

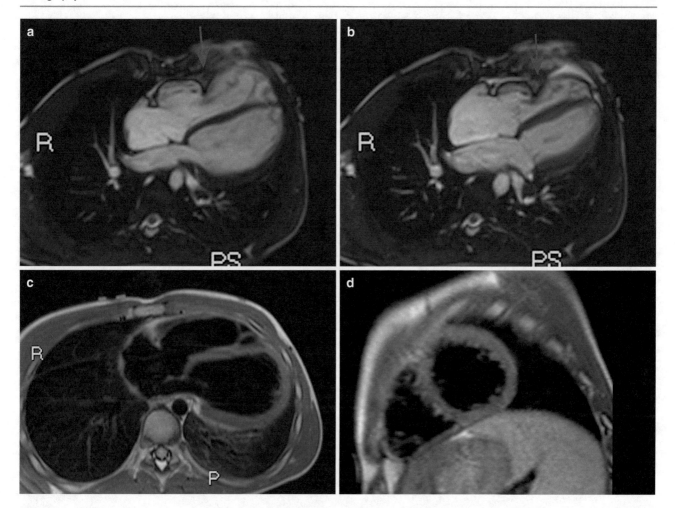

Fig. 6.19 Panels **a** and **b**: SSFP cine images in horizontal long axis. (**a**): End-diastolic frame; (**b**): end-systolic frame. The arrows show an indentation due presumably to the residual pericardial layer. Panels **c** and **d**: proton density-weighted images: (**c**) in horizontal long-axis and (**d**) in short-axis view. No apparent evidence of pericardium is detectable in correspondence of the lateral segments

Bibliography

1. Friedrich MG, Sechtem U, Schulz-Menger J, Holmvang G, Alakija P, Cooper LT, White JA, Abdel-Aty H, Gutberlet M, Prasad S, Aletras A, Laissy JP, Paterson I, Filipchuk NG, Kumar A, Pauschinger M, Liu P, International Consensus Group on Cardiovascular Magnetic Resonance in Myocarditis. Cardiovascular magnetic resonance in myocarditis: a JACC White Paper. J Am Coll Cardiol. 2009;53(17):1475–87.

2. Imazio M, Pedrotti P, Quattrocchi G, et al. Multimodality imaging of pericardial diseases. J Cardiovasc Med (Hagerstown). 2016;17:774–82.

3. Kumar A, Sato K, Yzeiraj E, et al. Quantitative pericardial delayed hyperenhancement informs clinical course in recurrent pericarditis. J Am Coll Cardiol Img. 2017;10:1337–46.

4. Alraies MC, AlJaroudi W, Yarmohammadi H, Yingchoncharoen T, Schuster A, Senapati A, Tariq M, Kwon D, Griffin BP, Klein AL. Usefulness of cardiac magnetic resonance-guided management in patients with recurrent pericarditis. Am J Cardiol. 2015;115(4):542–7.

5. Cremer PC, Tariq MU, Karwa A, Alraies MC, Benatti R, Schuster A, Agarwal S, Flamm SD, Kwon DH, Klein AL. Quantitative assessment of pericardial delayed hyperenhancement predicts clinical improvement in patients with constrictive pericarditis treated with anti-inflammatory therapy. Circ Cardiovasc Imaging. 2015;8(5):e003125.

6. Alraies MC, AlJaroudi W, Yarmo Hammadi H, Yingchoncharoen T, Schuster A, Senapati A, Tariq M, Kwon D, Griffin BP, Klein AL. Usefulness of cardiac magnetic resonance-guided management in patients with recurrent pericarditis. Am J Cardiol. 2015;115(4):542–7.

7. Lombardi M, Plein S, Petersen S, Bucciarelli-Ducci C, Valsangiacomo-Buechel M, Basso C, Ferrari V. The EACVI textbook of cardiovascular magnetic resonance. Oxford; Oxford University Press; 2018.

8. Vita T, Okada DR, Veillet-Chowdhury M, Bravo PE, Mullins E, Hulten E, Agrawal M, Madan R, Taqueti VR, Steigner M, Skali H, Kwong RY, Stewart GC, Dorbala S, Di Carli MF, Blankstein R. Complementary value of cardiac magnetic resonance imaging and positron emission tomography/computed tomography in the assessment of cardiac sarcoidosis. Circ Cardiovasc Imaging. 2018;11(1).

9. Moura-Ferreira S, Budts W, Bogaert J. Left pericardial congenital defect: the heart shows its moves at CMR. Eur Heart J Cardiovasc Imaging. 2017;18(11):1270.

7.1 Aortic Congenital Diseases

7.1.1 Aortic Double Arch

Medical History Female, 26 y.o. Surgical repair of inter-atrial defect at the age of 6 years and aortic valvular substitution with a stented biological prosthesis at the age of 16 years. Routine follow-up.

CMR Flowchart Stack of cine images in short-axis view to evaluate biventricular volumes and function. Cine images at the level of the prosthetic aortic valve. Cine images of thoracic aorta ("candy cane"). Angio 3D (CEMRA) of thoracic aorta.

Main CMR Findings Normal volumes and function of both ventricles. Normal position and function of the prosthetic aortic valve (Movie 7.1 and Movie 7.2). Unexpected double arch of the aorta (Movie 7.3).

Conclusion Favourable clinical evolution of previous surgical interventions. Unexpected double arch of the aorta.

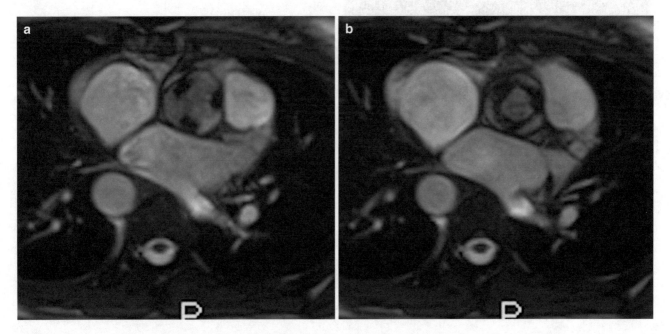

Fig. 7.1 (**a** and **b**) Cine images. Still frames in end diastole (**a**) and end systole (**b**) at the level of the aortic prosthetic valve

Electronic Supplementary Material The online version of this chapter (https://doi.org/10.1007/978-3-030-41830-4_7) contains supplementary material, which is available to authorized users.

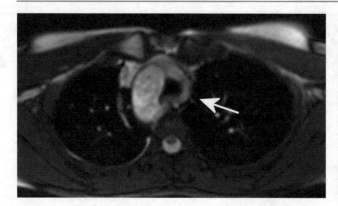

Fig. 7.2 Cine images in axial plane at the level of the aortic arch. Still frame. Evidence of double-aortic arch (arrow) with predominant right-sided aortic arch

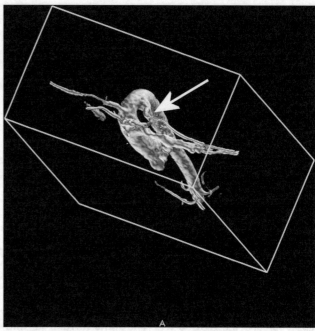

Fig. 7.4 Angio 3D CEMRA of thoracic aorta. The arrow shows the small left-sided aortic arch

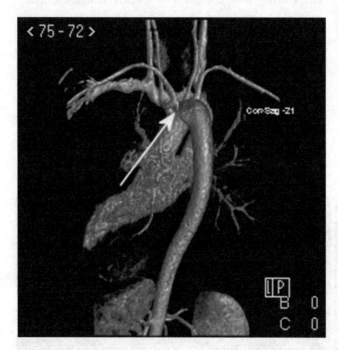

Fig. 7.3 Angio 3D CEMRA of thoracic aorta. The arrow shows the small left-sided aortic arch

7.1.2 Aortic Coarctation

Medical History Male, 13 y.o. Previous surgical correction of aortic coarctation and closure of patent Botallo oductus. Two previous percutaneous angioplasties because recurrence of aortic coarctation. Currently hypertension during effort. Annual follow-up.

CMR Flowchart Stack of cine images in short-axis view to evaluate biventricular volumes and function. Cine images in oblique plane to evaluate the ascending aorta, the aortic arch, and the descending aorta ("candy-cane" view). Flow images before and after the anatomic coarctation to evaluate the local flow amount. Angiography images (CEMRA) acquired during the injection of a bolus of contrast agent (0.2 mmol/kg). LGE images of the left ventricle.

Main CMR Findings Normal biventricular regional and global function. Normal thickness of left-ventricle walls. At cine images ("candy cane") evidence of reduced diameter at the isthmus level (Movie 7.4). Abnormal lack of decrease of the intra-aortic flow along the course of the vessel. At angiography evidence of recurrence of aortic coarctation at the isthmic level.

Conclusion Recurrence of aortic coarctation with intra-aortic pathologic flow.

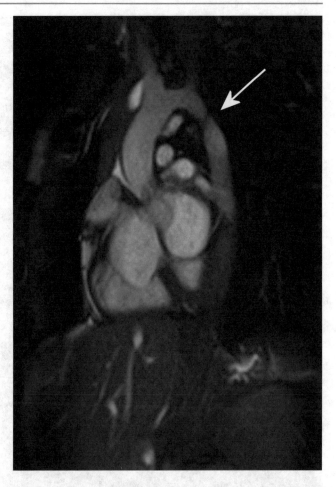

Fig. 7.5 Still frame from a cine SSFP sequence in oblique plane to obtain images from the thoracic aorta ("candy-cane" projection). Evidence of reduced diameter and loss of signal at the level of the isthmus (arrow)

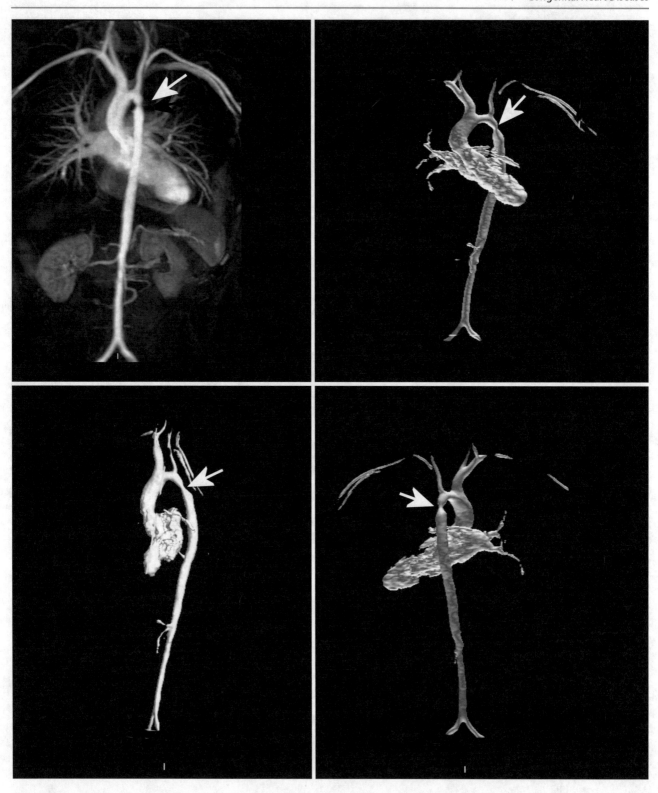

Fig. 7.6 3D images from a CEMRA sequence showing the isthmic coarctation (arrows). Left superior panel: 3D angiography, coronal view. Upper right panel and lower panels: volume rendering of the 3D volume and view from different projections

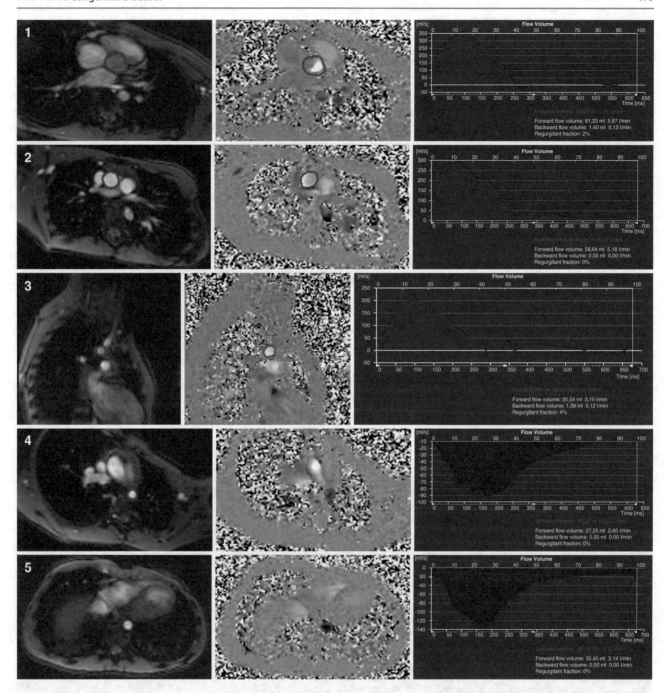

Fig. 7.7 Phase-contrast images (left panels: magnitude, middle panels: flow images) obtained at different levels of the aorta: (1) at the level of the aortic root (61.2 ml/beat), (2) at the level of the ascending aorta (58.6 ml/beat), (3) at the level of the aortic arch (35.5 ml/beat), (4) at the level of the stenotic isthmic region (27.2 ml/beat), (5) at the level of the diaphragm (35.4 ml/beat)

7.1.3 Stented Aortic Coarctation

Medical History Male, 17 y.o. Previous stenting of aortic coarctation. Annual follow-up.

CMR Flowchart Stack of cine images in short-axis view to evaluate biventricular volumes and function. Cine images in oblique plane to evaluate the ascending aorta, the aortic arch, and the descending aorta ("candy-cane" view). Flow images before and after the coarctation to evaluate the local flow amount. Angiographic images (CEMRA) acquired during the injection of a bolus of contrast agent (0.2 mmol/kg).

Main CMR Findings Normal biventricular regional and global function. Normal thickness of left-ventricle walls. At cine images ("candy cane") not the whole aorta is visible due to the tortuous course (Movie 7.5). Evidence of loss of signal at the level of the previous stenting. Normal decrease of the intra-aortic flow along the course. At angiography presence of large collateral connection.

Conclusion Turbulence of flow through the aortic coarctation previously stented. Normal flow values along the vessel. Favourable evolution of previous stenting.

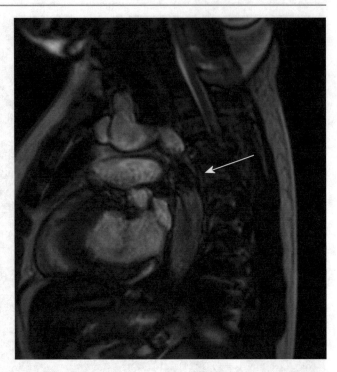

Fig. 7.8 Still frame from a cine SSFP sequence in oblique plane to obtain images from the stented region of the aorta. Evidence of loss of signal due to the presence of the metallic stent and the turbulence of flow

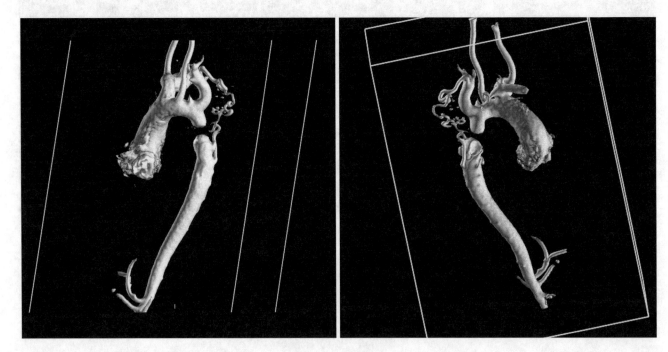

Fig. 7.9 3D images from a CEMRA sequence showing the loss of signal due to the metallic stent. Evidence of a large residual collateral vessel

7.1.4 Patent Ductus Arteriosus

Medical History Female, 79 y.o. Worsening dyspnea. Functional class III (NYHA).

CMR Flowchart Stack of cine images in short-axis view to evaluate biventricular volumes and function. SSFP images in oblique plane to identify the patent Ductus Arteriosus. Phase-contrast images to evaluate the aortic and pulmonary flow. Contrast-enhanced Magnetic Resonance Angiography (CEMRA) to assess the presence and location of the patent Ductus Arteriosus. LGE images acquired 10 min after c.a. administration (0.2 mmol/kg) to assess the presence of fibro-necrotic tissue within the myocardium.

Main CMR Findings Slight increase of left atrial and left ventricle volumes (Movie 7.6). Enlargement of Pulmonary trunk (Movie 7.7). Presence of patent Ductus Arteriosus (Movie 7.8 and Movie 7.9). Significant Sin>Dx shunt: Qp/Qs 0.62 (evaluated proximally to the Ductus Arteriosus).

Conclusion Patent Ductus Arteriosus.

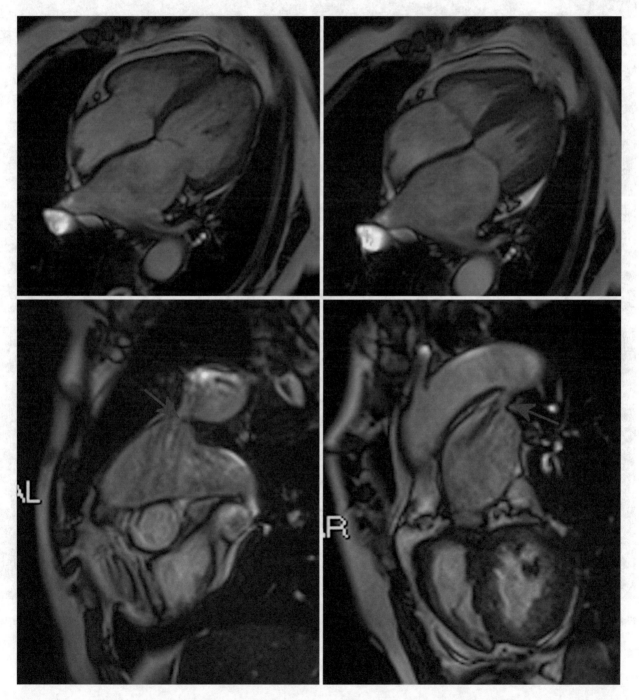

Fig. 7.10 SSFP cine images in horizontal long-axis (upper panels: end diastole on the left and end systole on the right) and in oblique views (lower panels). Evidence of slight increase of volumes of left atrium and left ventricle. Evidence in the oblique views of the patent Ductus Arteriosus (arrows) and turbulent flow within the Pulmonary trunk

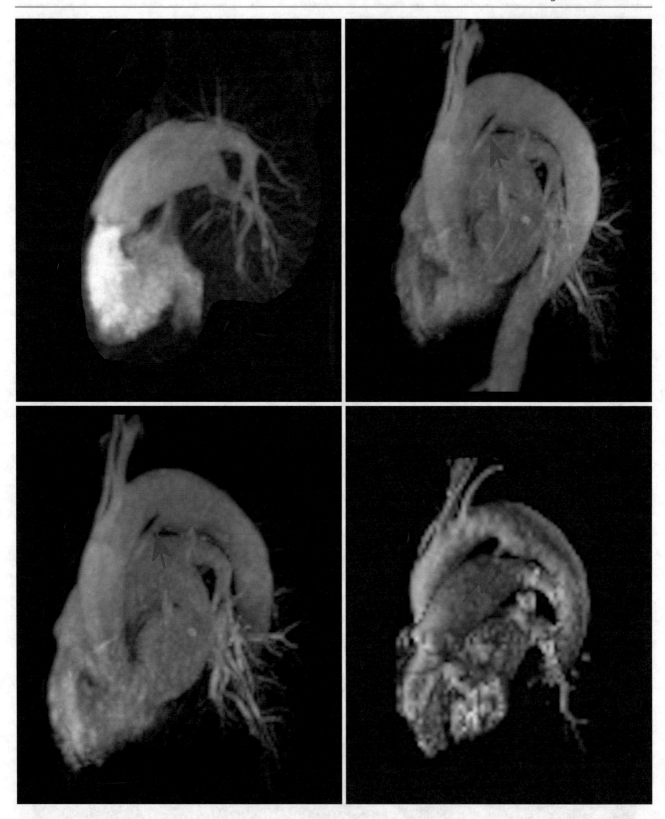

Fig. 7.11 Contrast-enhanced magnetic resonance angiography. Evidence of dilatation of the Pulmonary trunk. During the arterial phase evidence of the patent Ductus Arteriosus (arrows)

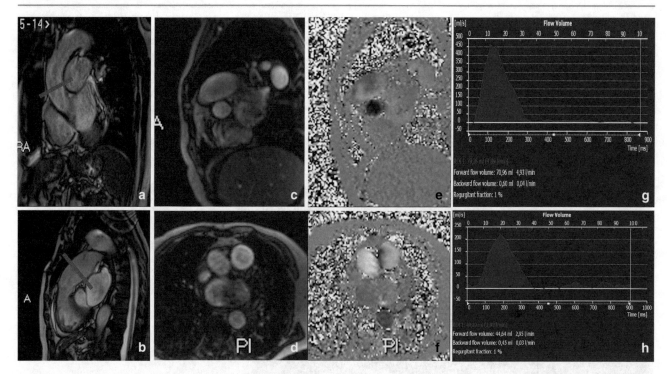

Fig. 7.12 Phase-contrast images obtained to measure the flow through the Aorta (upper panels) and through the Pulmonary Artery (lower panels) proximally to the Ductus Arteriosus (on the left panels); In panel **a** and **b** the red lines indicate the position utilized to obtain the phase-contrast images. In panel **c** and **d** the magnitudo images. In panel **e** and **f** the flow images. On the right panels (**g** and **h**) the final analysis of the flow images. The Qp/Qs resulted to be 0.60

7.1.5 Marfan Syndrome

Medical History Male, 11 y.o. Asymptomatic. Dilatation of aortic root at Echocardiography. Marfanoid appearance (160 cm × 31 kg).

CMR Flowchart Stack of SSFP cine images in short axis to evaluate the biventricular function. SSFP images in vertical and horizontal long axis to evaluate the mitral function. SSFP images in short axis of the aortic root, ascending aorta, aortic arch, and descending Aorta to evaluate the bidimensional diameters. Phase-contrast images at the level of the aortic valve to assess the presence/absence of valvular regurgitation. 3D contrast angiography (CEMRA) of thoracic Aorta to evaluate the course and the morphology of the vessel.

Main CMR Findings Pectus excavatum, normal biventricular function. Light dilatation of aortic root and ascending Aorta (Movie 7.10). Prolapse of both the mitral leaflets.

Conclusion Marfan syndrome: skeletal abnormalities, mitral prolapse, dilatation of the aortic root and of the ascending Aorta.

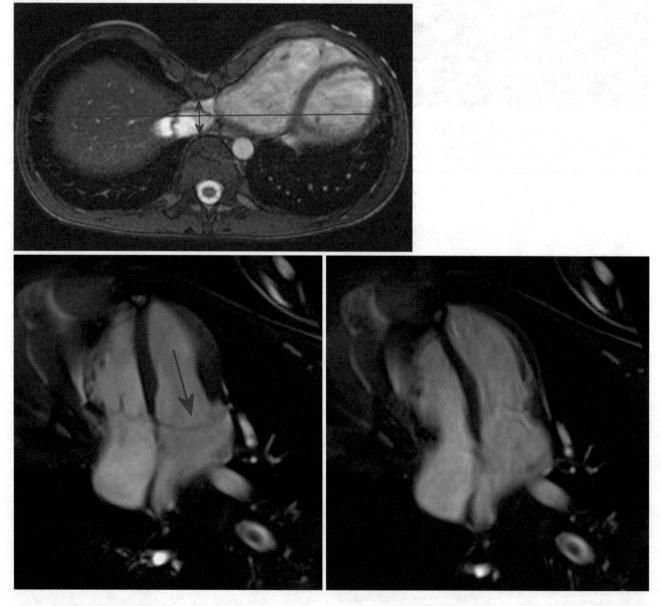

Fig. 7.13 Upper panel: Still frame from a SSFP cine sequence. Evidence of pectus excavatum and shift of the mediastinal mass toward the left side. Minimum anteroposterior distance of 3 cm. Haller index >9 (n.v. <2). Lower panels: Still frames from a SSFP cine sequence. Left panel: end-systolic frame. Right panel: end-diastolic frame. Evidence of mitral prolapse (arrow)

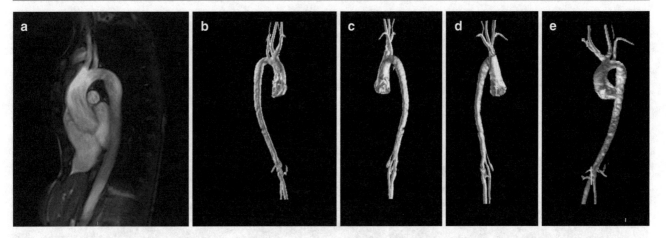

Fig. 7.14 Panel **a**: still frame from a cine sequence on sagittal plane. Panels **b–e**: images from a 3D contrast angiography. Evidence of dilatation of the aortic root and of ascending Aorta

7.1.6   Aortic Dissection in Marfan Syndrome

Clinical History Female, 51 y.o. Affected by Marfan syndrome. Previous substitution of aortic valve and ascending Aorta (Bentall procedure). Previous diagnosis of aortic dissection.

CMR Flowchart Stack of SSFP cine images in short axis to evaluate the biventricular function. SSFP images in sagittal plane and in local short-axis view of the thoracic Aorta to assess its course, dimensions, and morphology. SSFP cine images at the level of the aortic valve. Phase-contrast images at the level of the aortic valve. 3D contrast angiography (CEMRA) of the thoracic Aorta.

Main CMR Findings Presence os a large aneurism at the level of the diaphragmatic Aorta (60×81 mm, AP $\times$ LL) and chronic dissection of descending Aorta (Movie 7.11).

Conclusion Previous substitution of aortic valve and ascending Aorta (Bentall procedure). Aneurism and dissection of Aorta in Marfan syndrome.

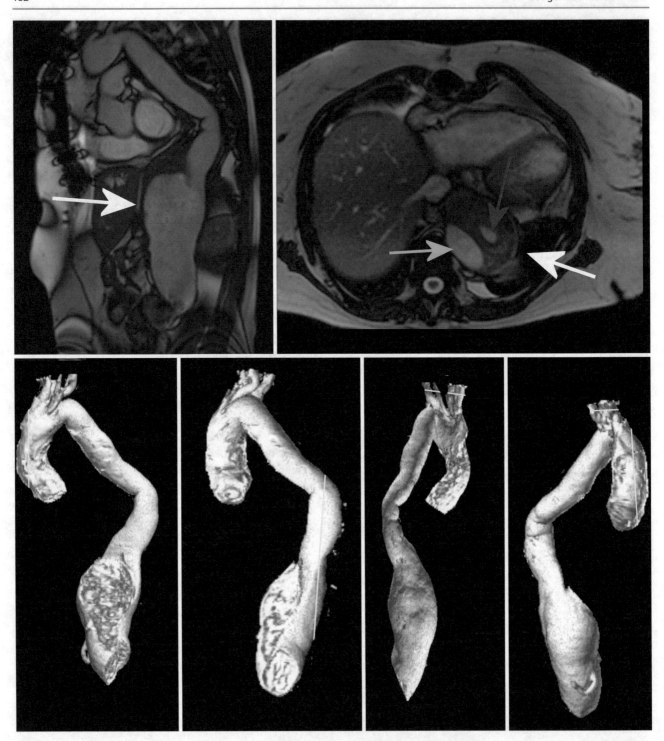

Fig. 7.15 Upper panels: SSFP cine images obtained in sagittal plane (left) and axial plane (right). Tortuous course of thoracic Aorta with diffuse abnormalities of the profile. Aneurism and dissection of the Aorta at the level of the diaphragm with evidence of thrombotic mate- rial partially filling the vessel and surrounding the true (green arrow) and the false (red arrow) lumen. Lower panels: four views of thoracic Aorta from a 3D contrast angiography with evidence of a large aneu- rism at the level of the thoracoabdominal part of the vessel

7.2 Anomalous Veno-Atrial Connection

7.2.1 Anomalous Veno-Atrial Connection with Partial Abnormal Venous Return

Clinical History 30-year-old male. Asymptomatic runner. At Echocardiography dilatation of the right ventricle in the presence of normal left ventricle. TAPSE: normal. Normal size of Inferior Vena Cava. Mild tricuspid regurgitation. Slight billowing of the posterior leaflet of the mitral valve with no evidence of significant regurgitation.

CMR Flowchart Stack of cine images in short-axis view to evaluate biventricular function, volumes, ventricular output, and Qp/Qs. Phase-contrast flow images at the level of ascending aorta and at the level of pulmonary artery for a precise evaluation of forward flow. Phase-contrast flow images at the level of superior and inferior vena cava to define the systemic and brachiocephalic venous return. 3D CEMRA angiography to define the connection between the venous structure and the atria. LGE images in long and short axis for characterization of myocardium.

Main CMR Findings Persistent Left Superior Vena Cava. Left upper Pulmonary Vein into Brachiocephalic Vein and a QP/Qs equal to 1.5. Moderate dilatation of the right heart (Movie 7.12): right-ventricle volume: 122 ml/m^2 with preserved systolic function. Normal sizes, volumes, and systolic function of the left ventricle.

Small area of uptake of contrast media at the level of inferior junction between right-ventricle free wall and left ventricle, with no pathologic meaning.

Conclusion Anomalous partial pulmonary venous return. Persistent Left Superior Vena Cava. Surgeon consultation recommended.

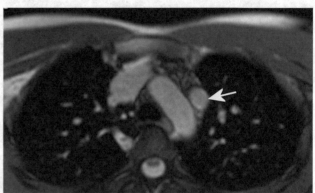

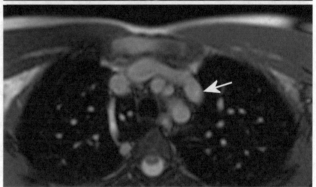

Fig. 7.16 SSFP cine images. Still frame. Axial plane. Upper panel image at the level of the aortic arch. The arrow shows the abnormal pulmonary vein. In the lower panel the abnormal connection between the Pulmonary Vein and the Brachiocephalic Trunk (arrow)

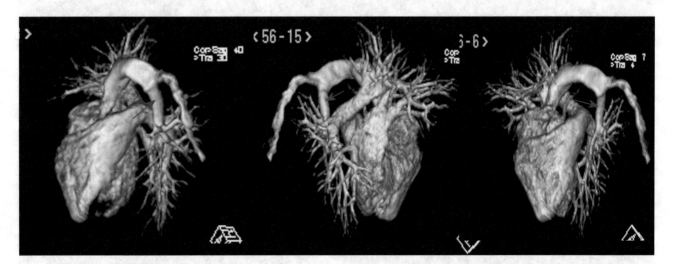

Fig. 7.17 Contrast-enhanced magnetic resonance angiography (CEMRA) showing the presence of an abnormal large pulmonary vein originating from the lower portion of the left lung. Three views of the abnormal vein. The arrows show the connection between the abnormal vessel and the Brachiocephalic Trunk

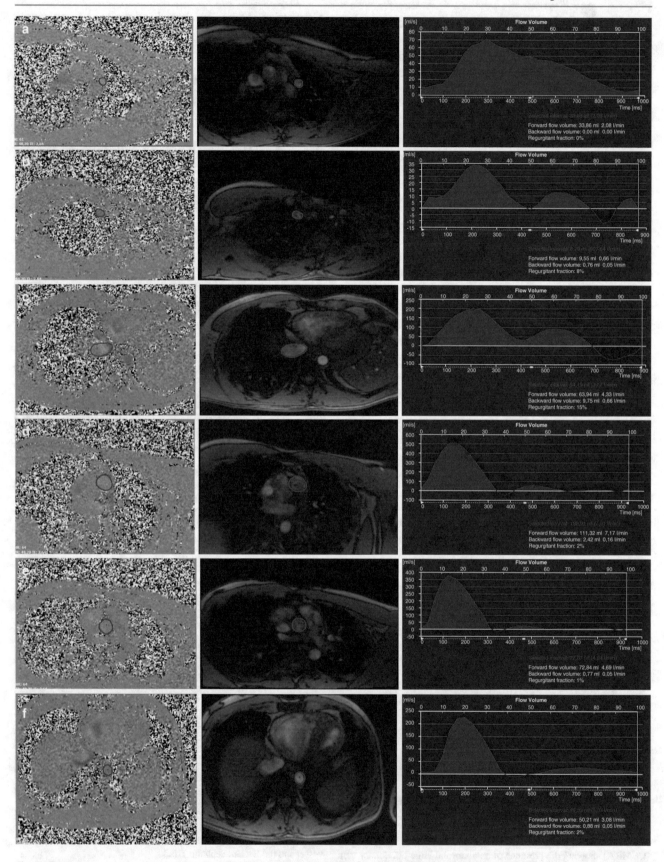

Fig. 7.18 Left panels: phase-contrast images; middle panels: magnitude images; right panels: measurement of flows within the region of interest as shown in the magnitude and phase-contrast images. (**a**) Persistent Left Superior Vena Cava, (**b**) Right Superior Vena Cava, (**c**) Inferior Vena Cava, (**d**) Pulmonary Artery, (**e**) Ascending Aorta, (**f**) Aorta at the level of diaphragm

7.2.2 Abnormal Veno-Atrial Connection, Left>Right Shunt

Medical History Female, 38 y.o. Previous stroke. Previous closure of interatrial defect. Recent episode of transient diplopia.

CMR Flowchart Stack of cine images in short-axis view to evaluate biventricular volumes and function. Stack of cine images in para-axial plane to evaluate the connection of pulmonary veins and right atrium, and superior and inferior Vena Cava. Black blood images to obtain images at the level of veno-atrial connection. Phase-contrast images to evaluate the flow at the level of the ascending Aorta and the Pulmonary Trunk.

Three-dimensional contrast-enhanced angiography (CEMRA) performed during the injection of contrast agent (0.2 mmol/kg) followed by LGE images.
Severe Sin>Dx shunt with a Qp/Qs = 3.45.

Main CMR Findings Left-ventricle volume within the normal limits with preserved global function (EF 64%). Right-ventricle dilatation (ED 211 ml/m^2, ES 81 ml/m^2). Evidence in all set of images of an anomalous connection of right pulmonary veins to the superior Vena Cava just above the right atrium (Movie 7.13).

Conclusion Abnormal veno-atrial connection with severe sin>dx shunt. Surgeon consultation recommended.

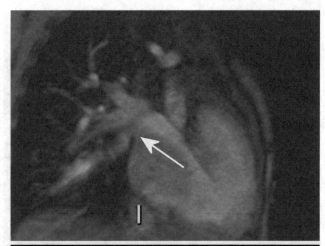

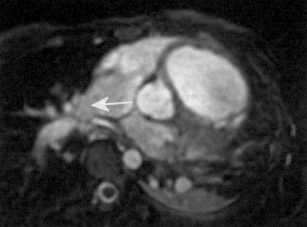

Fig. 7.19 Cine images in coronal view (upper panel) and in axial plane lower panel at the level of the anomalous connection of the right pulmonary veins into the superior Vena Cava, just above the right atrium (arrows)

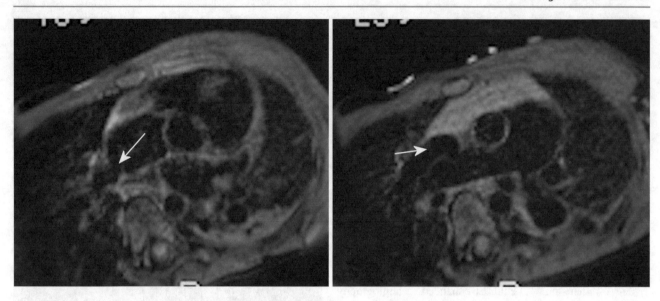

Fig. 7.20 Black blood images in oblique planes at the level of the anomalous connection (arrows)

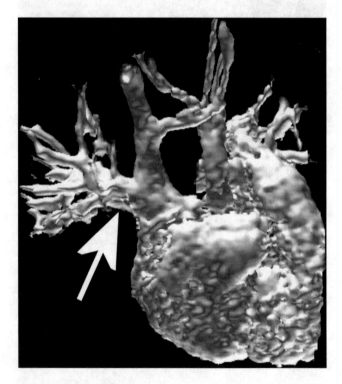

Fig. 7.21 Three-dimensional contrast agent angiography (CEMRA). Evidence of the anomalous connection between the right pulmonary veins and the superior Vena Cava

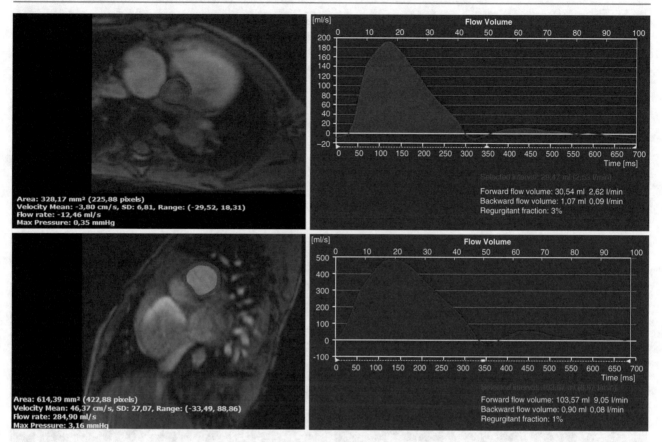

Fig. 7.22 Phase-contrast images at the level of the ascending aorta (upper panels) and at the level of the Pulmonary Trunk (lower panels). Magnitude images (left panels) and results of the flow analysis (right panels)

7.2.3 Scimitar Syndrome

Medical History Female, 19 y.o. Palpitation. At Echocardiography enlargement of right ventricle.

CMR Flowchart Stack of cine images in short-axis view to evaluate biventricular volumes and function. Stack of SSFP cine images in axial planes to assess the venous-atrial connection. Phase-contrast images at the level of the ascending Aorta and at the level of the Pulmonary Trunk to evaluate the Qp/Qs. 3D contrast angiography (CEMRA).

Main CMR Findings Right-ventricle volume at upper limits (EDV 93 ml/m²) with preserved global function. Abnormal right pulmonary vein connected to the inferior Vena Cava. Hypoplastic right lung. Pathologic Qp/Qs: 1.5.

Conclusion Partial anomalous venous connection and hypoplastic right lung. Scimitar syndrome.

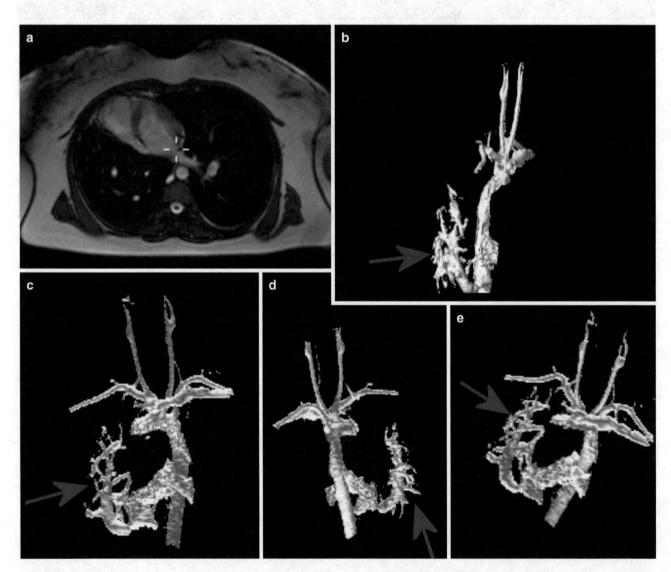

Fig. 7.23 Panel **a**: Still frame from SSFP cine sequence in axial plane showing a hypoplastic right lung, with the mediastinal mass shifted toward the right side. Panels **b–e**: four views from 3D contrast angiography showing the anomalous vein draining into the inferior Vena Cava (arrows). Images provided by Dr. Lorenzo Monti, Humanitas Research Hospital, Rozzano, Milan, Italy

7.2.4 Cor Triatriatum

Medical History Male, 62 y.o. Palpitations. Hypertension. At Echocardiography membranous structure within an enlarged left atrium.

CMR Flowchart Stack of cine images in short-axis view to evaluate biventricular volumes and function. Stack of SSFP cine images in horizontal long axis. SSFP cine images and Black Blood PD images in three-chamber view and in oblique plane to evaluate the membranous structure within the left atrium.

Main CMR Findings Normal biventricular volumes and function. Increased thickness of left-ventricle walls. Presence of a mobile membranous structure within the left atrium. The left atrium is divided into two chambers widely communicating (Movie 7.14, Movie 7.15 and Movie 7.16).

Conclusion Cor triatriatum.

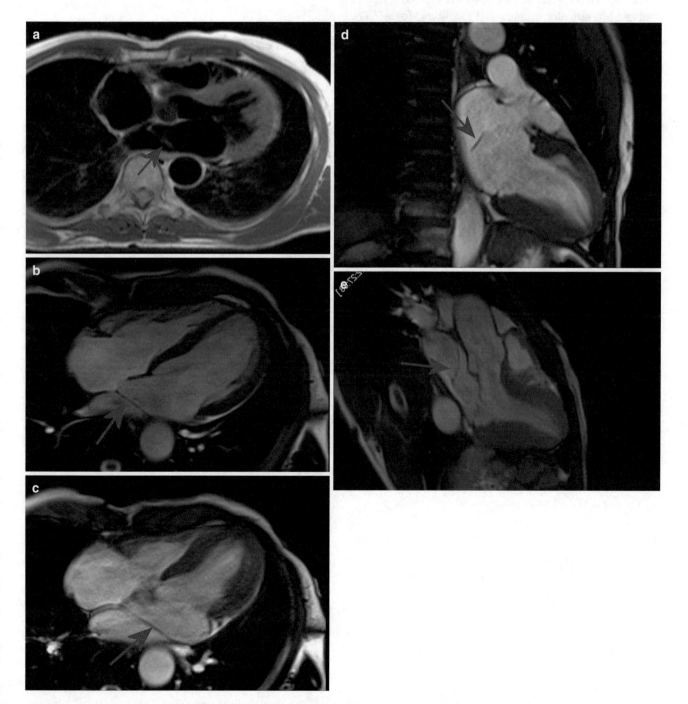

Fig. 7.24 Panel **a**: PDw image in oblique plane. Panel **b**: SSFP still frame from a cine sequence in horizontal long axis. Panel **c**: SSFP still frame from a cine sequence in oblique plane. Panel **d**: SSFP still frame from a cine sequence. In vertical long-axis view. Panel **e**: SSFP still frame from a cine sequence in three-chamber view. Evidence of a tiny membrane dividing the atrium into two chambers (arrows)

7.3   Complex Congenital Heart Diseases

7.3.1   Tetralogy of Fallot

Medical History Female, 48 y.o. Asymptomatic. Postsurgical status (surgical intervention at the age of 8 years). Echocardiographic and hemodynamic evidence of subvalvular pulmonary stenosis. Unsuccessful attempt of positioning a transcatheter pulmonary valve (too large diameter!!).

CMR Flowchart Stack of cine images in short-axis view to evaluate biventricular volumes and function (Movie 7.17). Cine images in oblique view to obtain diagnostic images at the level of the right outflow tract (Movie 7.18). Phase-contrast images at the level of the Pulmonary Trunk and at the level of the left and right Pulmonary Artery, and at the level of the ascending Aorta to calculate the Qp/Qs ratio. Contrast-enhanced three-dimensional angiography (CEMRA) (Movie 7.19). Postcontrast LGE images (GRE-IR).

Main CMR Findings Left-ventricle volume and global function normal. Significant enlargement of right ventricle (RVEDV 143 ml/m², RVESV 66 ml/m², and preserved global function (EF 54%)). Dysplastic pulmonary valve with severe regurgitation. Right aortic arch. Persistent left superior Vena Cava.

Conclusion Post-surgical status of Fallot Tetralogy. Subvalvular pulmonary stenosis.

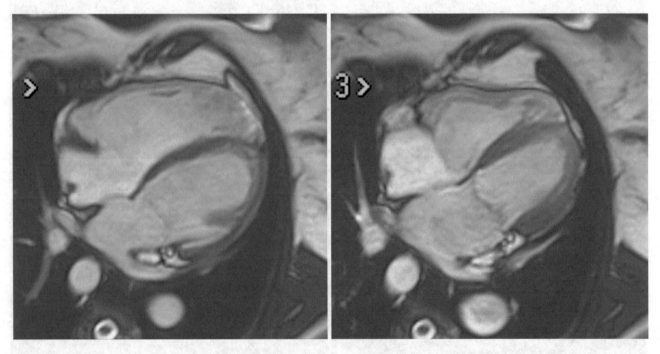

Fig. 7.25 SSFP cine images in horizontal long axis of the heart. Evidence of enlarged right ventricle. Left panel: end-diastolic frame. Right panel: end-systolic frame

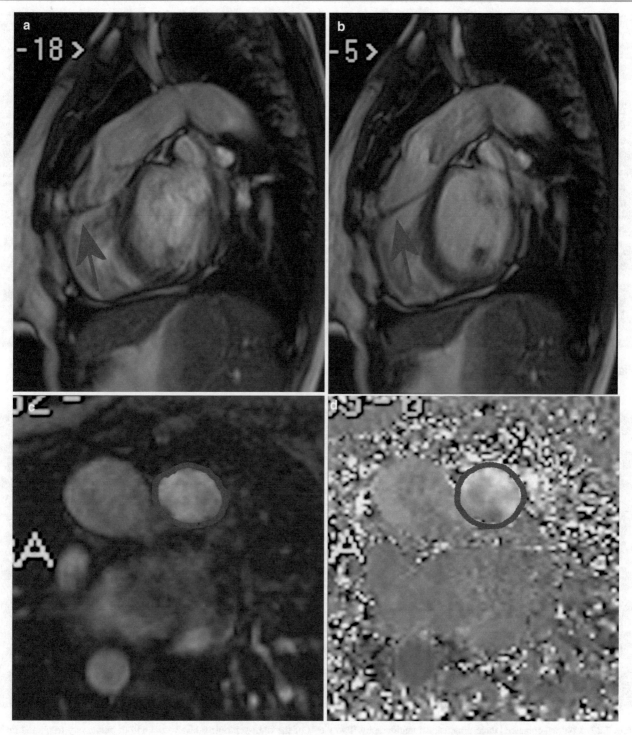

Fig. 7.26 Upper panels: SSFP cine images in oblique view to assess the right-ventricle outflow tract and the Pulmonary valve. Evidence of subvalvular stenosis (arrows), enlarged pulmonary valvular plane, and severe valvular regurgitation. (**a**) Systolic frame; (**b**) diastolic frame. Mid panels: phase-contrast images: (**c**) magnitude image; (**d**) flow image. In (**e**): the deriving flow scheme

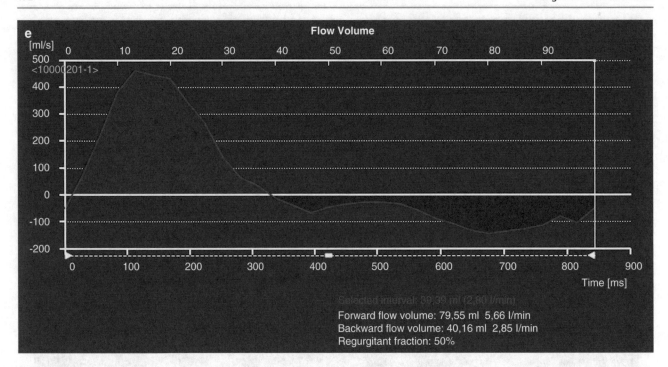

Flow Volume

Forward flow volume: 79,55 ml 5,66 l/min
Backward flow volume: 40,16 ml 2,85 l/min
Regurgitant fraction: 50%

Fig. 7.26 (continued)

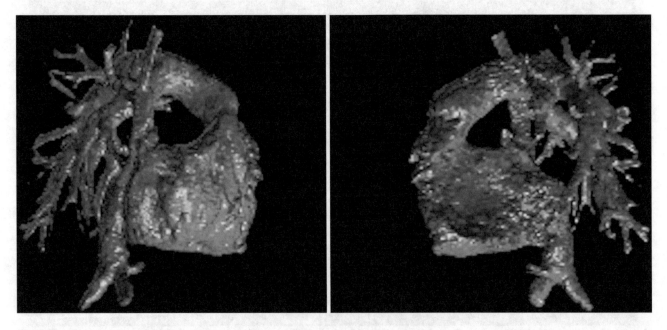

Fig. 7.27 Contrast-enhanced three-dimensional angiography. Two views of the right-ventricle outflow tract and of pulmonary trunk and main branches. (Left panel anterior view, right panel lateral view)

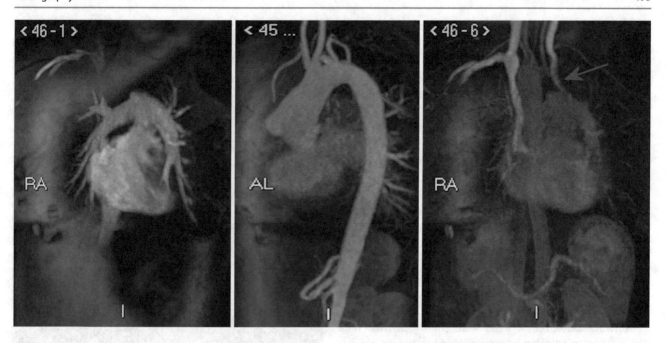

Fig. 7.28 Time-resolved contrast-enhanced three-dimensional angiography. Three consecutive three-dimensional acquisition volumes. Left panel: during the right section phase. Central panel: during the arterial phase. Right panel: during the venous phase. The arrow shows the persistence of the left superior vena cava

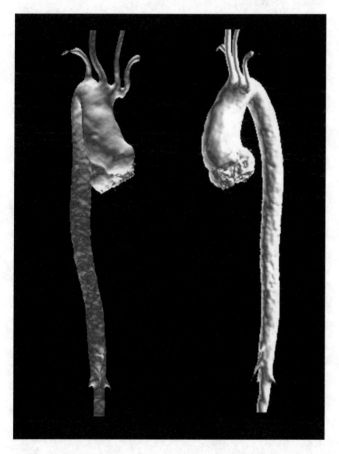

Fig. 7.29 Contrast-enhanced three-dimensional angiography. Two views of the arterial phase

7.3.2 Postsurgical Atrio-pulmonary Fontan Status

Medical History Female, 25 y.o. Affected by tricuspid atresia, hypoplastic right ventricle, ventricular septal defect, and pulmonary stenosis. She underwent fenestrated atrio-pulmonary Fontan intervention at the age of 3 years. Percutaneous closure of the fenestration at the age of 4 years. Recent palpitations and electrocardiographic evidence of ventricular tachycardia.

CMR Flowchart Stack of cine images in short-axis view to evaluate ventricular volumes and function. Contrast-enhanced 3D angiography (CEMRA) of the thoracic Aorta. LGE images to detect myocardial fibrosis.

Main CMR Findings Preserved ventricular function. Severely dilated right atrium with "smoke effect" and thrombotic stratification on the atrial wall. Dilated inferior Vena Cava. Patent connection between the atrium and the pulmonary arteries (Movie 7.20 and Movie 7.21). Hypoplastic right ventricle (Movie 7.22 and Movie 7.23). Mild flow acceleration through the aortic valve and mild aortic regurgitation. Right hemidiaphragmatic relaxation.

Conclusion Atrio-pulmonary Fontan circulation with severely dilated right atrium with thrombotic stratification on the atrial wall. Preserved ventricular function.

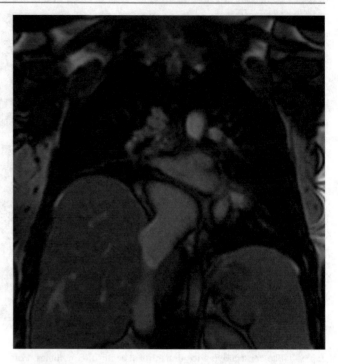

Fig. 7.30 SSFP still frame in coronal view. Right hemidiaphragmatic relaxation. Right-lung hypoplasia. Evidence of inferior Vena Cava dilatation. Liver is enlarged

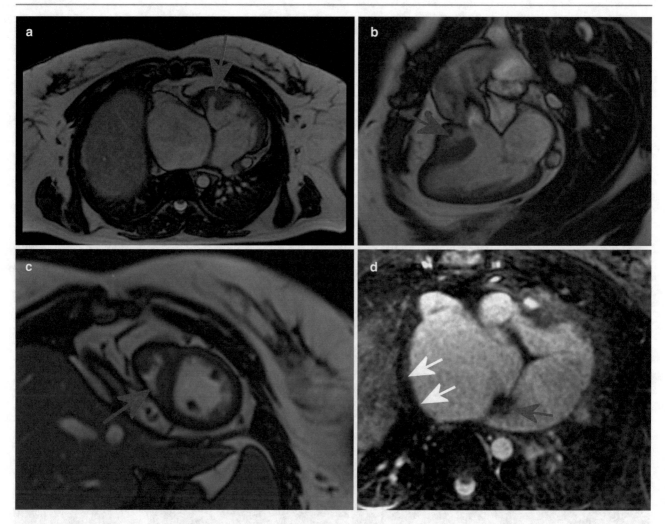

Fig. 7.31 Panel **a**: still frame from SSFP cine sequence in horizontal long axis. Evidence of a dilated right atrium. Hypoplastic right ventricle (red arrow). Panel **b**: still frame from SSFP cine sequence in vertical long axis. Evidence of a hypoplastic right ventricle (red arrow) communicating with the left ventricle through a ventricular septal defect. Panel **c**: still frame from SSFP cine sequence in short-axis view.

Evidence of a hypoplastic right ventricle (red arrow). Panel **d**: LGE image in horizontal long-axis view. Evidence of a metallic device occluding the postsurgical interatrial communication (red arrow). Enlarged right atrium with evidence of stratified thrombotic material (white arrows)

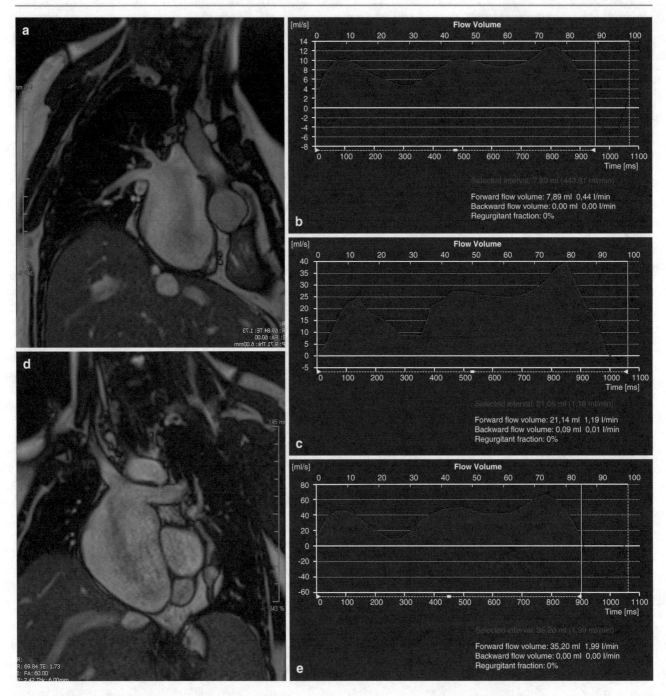

Fig. 7.32 Panel **a**: still frame from a SSFP cine sequence in oblique view showing the two right pulmonary connections with the right atrium and the relative measurement of flows (panels **b** and **c**). Panel **d**: still frame from a SSFP cine sequence in oblique view showing the superior vena cava draining to the right atrium (on the left side) and the left pulmonary artery connected to the right atrium (on the right side) with the relative measurement of flow (panel **e**)

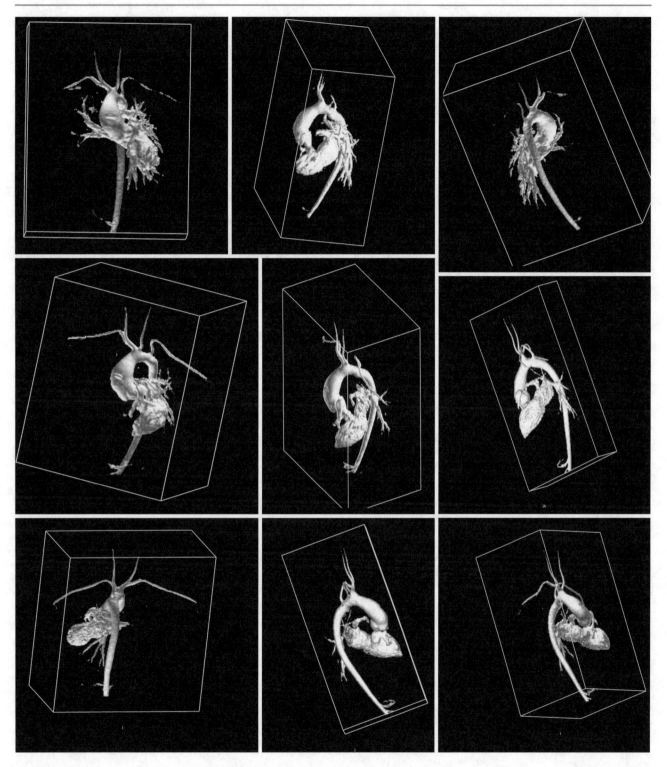

Fig. 7.33 Nine views from a three-dimensional contrast angiography showing the venous pulmonary connection with the left atrium, the ventricle, and the Aorta

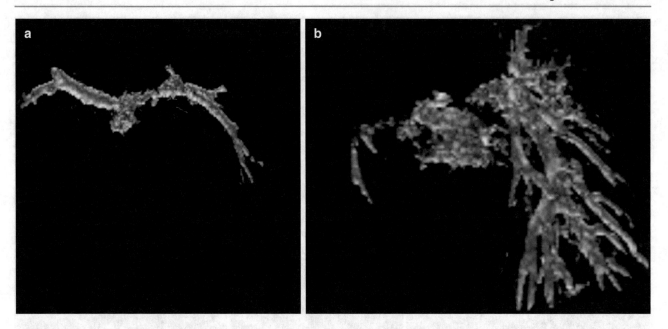

Fig. 7.34 Two views from a three-dimensional contrast angiography showing the left and right pulmonary connection with the right atrium (panel **a**). Evidence of a marked hypoplasia of the right-lung pulmonary arterial structure (panel **b**)

Bibliography

1. Lombardi M, Plein S, Petersen S, Bucciarelli-Ducci C, Valsangiacomo-Buechel M, Basso C, Ferrari V. The EACVI textbook of cardiovascular magnetic resonance. Oxford: Oxford University Press; 2018.
2. Ojaghi Haghigh Z, Sadeghpour A, Alizadehasl A. Isolated right sided anomalous pulmonary venous connection associated with significant right ventricular enlargement and intact interatrial septum. J Cardiovasc Thorac Res. 2012;4(4):123–4.
3. Sormani P, Roghi A, Cereda A, Peritore A, Milazzo A, Quattrocchi G, Giannattasio C, Pedrotti P. Partial anomalous pulmonary venous return as rare cause of right ventricular dilation: a retrospective analysis. Congenit Heart Dis. 2016;11(4):365–8.
4. Valsangiacomo-Buechel E, Muthurangu V. Congenital heart disease. In: Lombardi M, Plein S, Petersen S, Bucciarelli-Ducci C, Valsangiacoo Buechel M, Basso C, Ferrari V, editors. The EACVI textbook of cardiovascular magnetic resonance. Oxford: Oxford University Press; 2018.
5. Chen SS, Dimopoulos K, Alonso-Gonzalez R, Liodakis E, Teijeira-Fernandez E, Alvarez-Barredo M, Kempny A, Diller G, Uebing A, Shore D, Swan L, Kilner PJ, Gatzoulis MA, Mohiaddin RH. Prevalence and prognostic implication of restenosis or dilatation at the aortic coarctation repair site assessed by cardiovascular MRI in adult patients late after coarctation repair. Int J Cardiol. 2014;173(2):209–15.
6. Muzzarelli S, Meadows AK, Ordovas KG, Higgins CB, Meadows JJ. Usefulness of cardiovascular magnetic resonance imaging to predict the need for intervention in patients with coarctation of the aorta. Am J Cardiol. 2012;109(6):861–5.
7. Dormand H, Mohiaddin RH. Cardiovascular magnetic resonance in Marfan syndrome. J Cardiovasc Magn Reson. 2013;15:33.

Miscellanea

8.1 Pectus Excavatum

Clinical History Fifty-three-year-old female patient. In the past episodes of syncope. In 2014 admitted to ER because of acute chest pain. Evidence of normal coronary arteries.

CMR Flowchart Stack of cine images in short-axis view to evaluate biventricular volumes and function. Cine images and black blood PDw images in axial planes through the mediastinum. LGE images 10 min after a bolus of contrast agent (0.2 mmol/kg).

Main CMR Findings Evidence of pectus excavatum with a minimal distance between the thoracic vertebral body and the posterior face of the sternum of 39 mm and a Haller index (ratio between anteroposterior and lateral-lateral diameter) of 6 (normal value <2.5) (Movie 8.1).

Normal left ventricle size, volumes, and function.

Right-ventricle size and volumes are normal with the presence of systolic bulging in the lateral wall mid segment probably due to the abnormal shape of the thorax (Movie 8.2). No myocardial fibrosis in LGE images.

Conclusion Pectus excavatum with displacement of the mediastinum.

Electronic Supplementary Material The online version of this chapter (https://doi.org/10.1007/978-3-030-41830-4_8) contains supplementary material, which is available to authorized users.

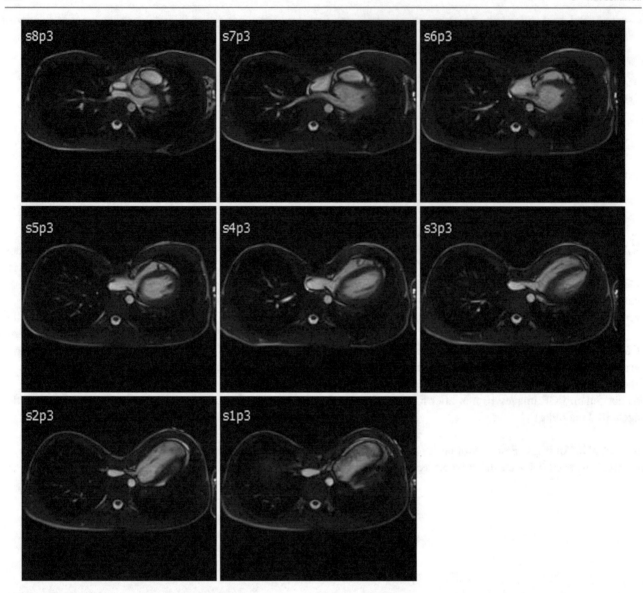

Fig. 8.1 Still frames from a SSFP cine sequence. Stack of images in axial projection. Evidence of displacement of the mediastinum and reduced distance between the sternum and the vertebral body

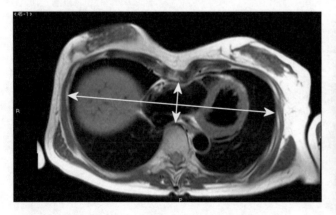

Fig. 8.2 Black blood images PDw. Axial projection. Minimal distance between the posterior sternal face and the vertebral body 3.9 cm. The latero-lateral diameter resulting in 21 cm

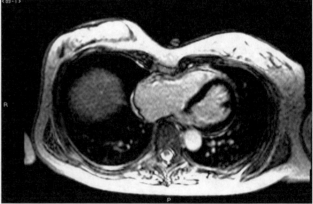

Fig. 8.3 LGE image. No evidence of myocardial or pericardial fibrosis

8.2 Coronary Fistula

Medical History Female, 17 y.o. Multiple venous malformations at skin level. ECG abnormalities. Presence of an extracardiac mass at the level of the apex.

CMR Flowchart Stack of cine images in short-axis view to evaluate biventricular volumes and function. Cine images in axial and oblique planes to identify the mass and its effect on the cardiac kinetic. Black blood T2w images. Black blood T1w images before and after the injection of a bolus of contrast agent (0.2 mmol/kg). LGE images.

Main CMR Findings Moderate reduction of left-ventricle global function (EF 49%). Evidence of a large extracardiac mass (71 × 50 × 31 mm (SI × AP × LL)) positioned from the lateral part of the left ventricle toward the right-ventricle free wall (Movie 8.3, Movie 8.4 and Movie 8.5). The mass appears isointense in T1w and hyperintense in T2w images. In T1w images signal intensity markedly increased after the injection of contrast agent. Inhomogeneous uptake in LGE images. No infiltrative behavior of the mass.

Conclusion The morphologic characteristics and the signal behavior as well as the uptake of contrast agent are compatible with a angiomatous mass as well as a coronary fistula. The latter resulting in the correct diagnosis after angiography.

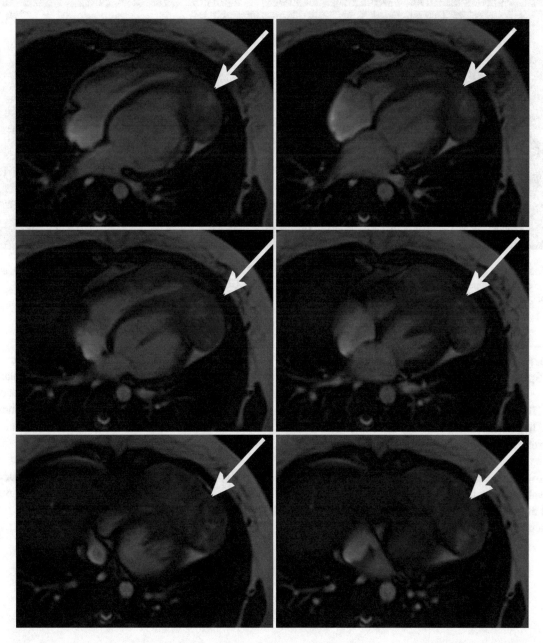

Fig. 8.4 SSFP cine images from three parallel planes in horizontal long axis. Left panels: end-diastolic frames. Right panels: end-systolic frames. The arrows show the para-cardiac mass and the relationship with the myocardium

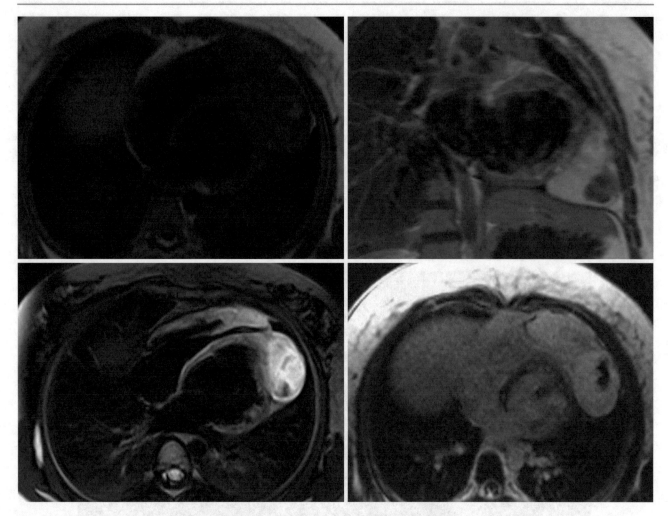

Fig. 8.5 Four images of the para-cardiac mass obtained with a black blood T1w sequence (upper left panel, axial plane); black blood T1w image (oblique plane) after the administration of contrast agent (0.2 mmol/kg), black blood T2w image (lower left panel, axial plane), and LGE image (lower right panel, axial plane)

8.3   Interventricular Septal Defect Spontaneously Closed

Clinical History 66-year-old female patient with a history of arterial hypertension and a history of ventricular extrasystoles. Normal Echocardiography.

CMR Flowchart Stack of SSFP cine images in short-axis view to evaluate biventricular function, segmental wall thickness, and myocardial mass. LGE images for myocardial tissue characterization.

Main CMR Findings Normal biventricular function. Evidence of a small diverticulum within the muscular interventricular septum (Movie 8.6). At LGE images presence of focal uptake of c.a. in correspondence of the diverticulum. No evidence of shunt in cine images. Qp/Qs = 1 evaluated by stroke volumes.

MR Report Conclusion Normal sizes, volumes, and function of left and right ventricles. Spontaneous closure of the interventricular muscular defect.

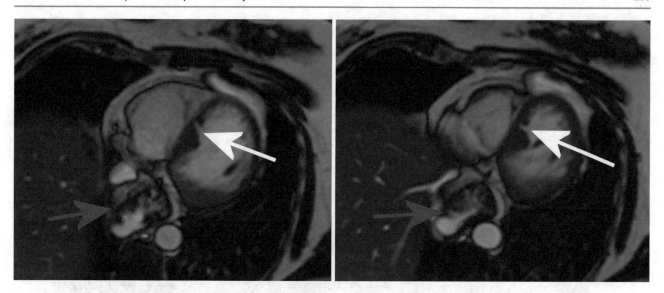

Fig. 8.6 SSFP cine images. Left panel: end-diastolic frame. Right panel: mid-systolic frame. The white arrows show the deep interventricular diverticulum without evidence of shunt. The red arrows show, as incidental finding, a large hiatus hernia

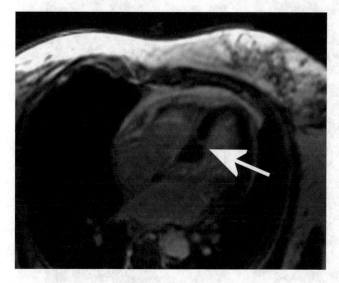

Fig. 8.7 LGE image showing the deep septal diverticulum focal fibrosis at the bottom

8.4 Abnormal Course of Coronary Arteries

Medical History Male, 43-year-old patient affected by transposition of great arteries and previous intervention of atrial switch.

CMR Flowchart The protocol focused on the detection of abnormalities in origin and proximal course of coronary arteries is limited to a 3D free-breathing whole-heart sequence.

Main CMR Findings Coronary arteries originating from posterior sinuses. Evidence of a long left main with a retropulmonary course originating together with the right coronary artery. A large marginal artery originates from the other posterior sinus.

Conclusion Anomalous origin and course of coronary arteries in a patient with a transposition of great arteries.

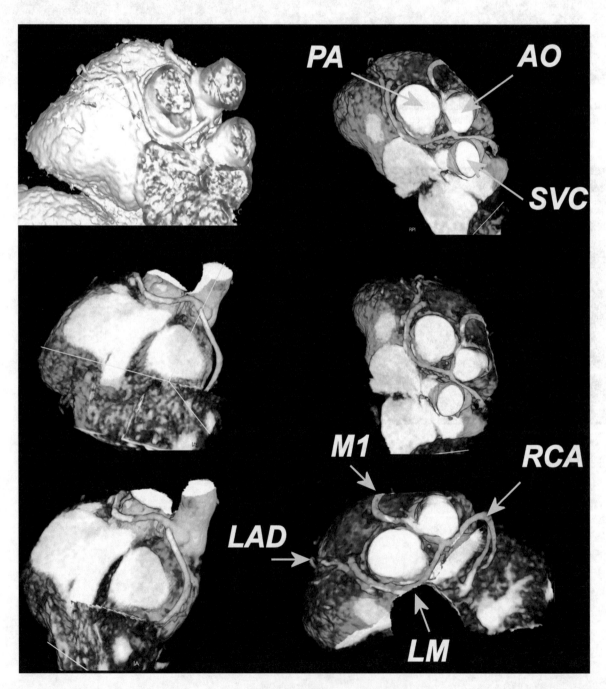

Fig. 8.8 3D free-breathing T2 prep whole-heart sequence. Left upper panel: the original 3D whole-heart volume. The other images are obtained after applying a volume-rendering algorithm and cutting part of the heart and vessels to enhance the course of the coronary arteries. *PA* Pulmonary Artery, *AO* Aorta, *SVC* Superior Vena Cava, *RCA* Right Coronary Artery, *LM* Left Main, *LAD* Left Anterior Descending Artery, *M1* Marginal Branch

8.5 Coronary Involvement in Kawasaki Disease

Medical History Male, 26 y.o. Diagnosis of Kawasaki disease at the age of 6. Asymptomatic.

CMR Flowchart Stack of cine images in images in in short-axis view to evaluate biventricular volumes and function. 3D free-breathing coronary angiography. Perfusion images during adenosine infusion. LGE images.

Main CMR Findings Left-ventricle volume and global function normal. Dilated proximal left anterior descending artery. No stress perfusion abnormalities (Movie 8.7 and Movie 8.8). No myocardial scar.

Conclusion Coronary involvement in Kawasaki disease. No inducible ischemia.

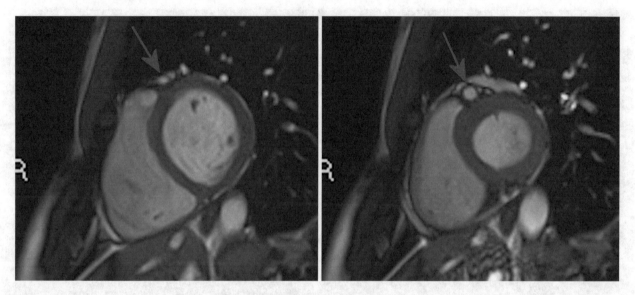

Fig. 8.9 SSFP cine images in short axis. Evidence of dilated coronary artery (proximal LAD) (arrows) which is more evident during the systolic phase (right panel) rather than during the diastolic frame (left panel). The cross-sectional diameter resulted to be 12 mm (max), unchanged with respect to the previous control (2 years earlier)

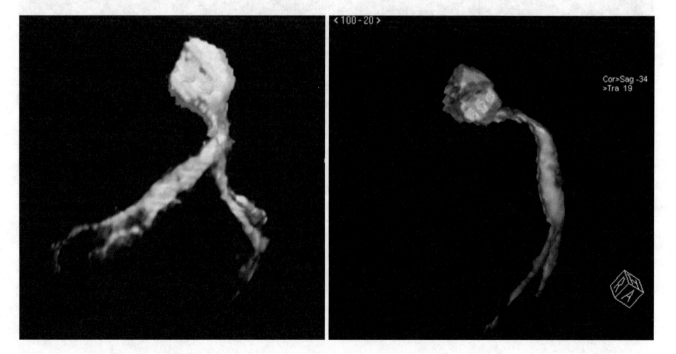

Fig. 8.10 Three-dimensional angiography, obtained in free breathing using navigator technique. Reconstruction and volume rendering of the left anterior descending artery with evidence of enlargement of the proximal section of the vessel

8.6   Chiari Network

Medical History Male, 57 y.o. Asymptomatic. At Echocardiography Evidence of an indefinite mass within the right atrium.

CMR Flowchart Stack of cine images in short-axis view to evaluate biventricular volumes and function. Cine images in oblique view to obtain diagnostic images at the level of the right atrium. T1w and T2w to characterize the intra-atrial mass.

Main CMR Findings Left-ventricle volume and global function normal. Cine images in oblique views show an elongated, irregular structure which is connected with the Eustachian valve at the inferior level and reaches the atrial roof (Movie 8.9, Movie 8.10 and Movie 8.11). The structure shows undefined signal characteristics.

Conclusion Chiari network.

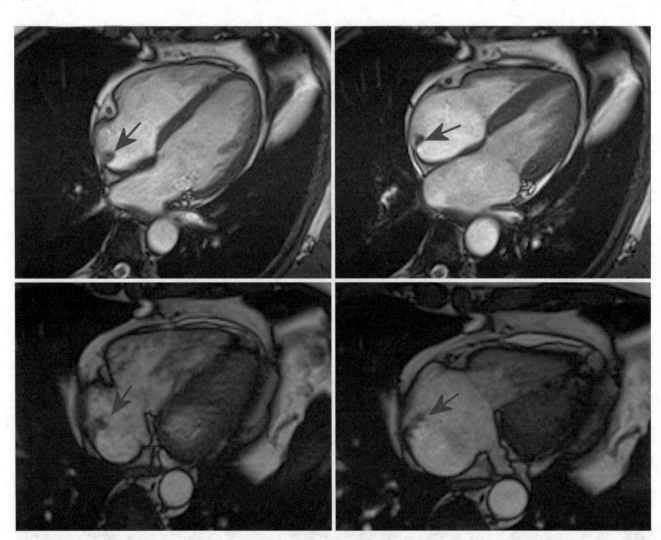

Fig. 8.11 SSFP cine images in horizontal long-axis (upper panels) and in oblique views (lower panels). The arrows show the presence of a mass at the level of the Eustachian valve. In the lower panels, obtained in oblique view the irregular shape is more evident in the end-systolic frame (right panel) (Left panels: end-diastolic frames; right panels: end-systolic frame)

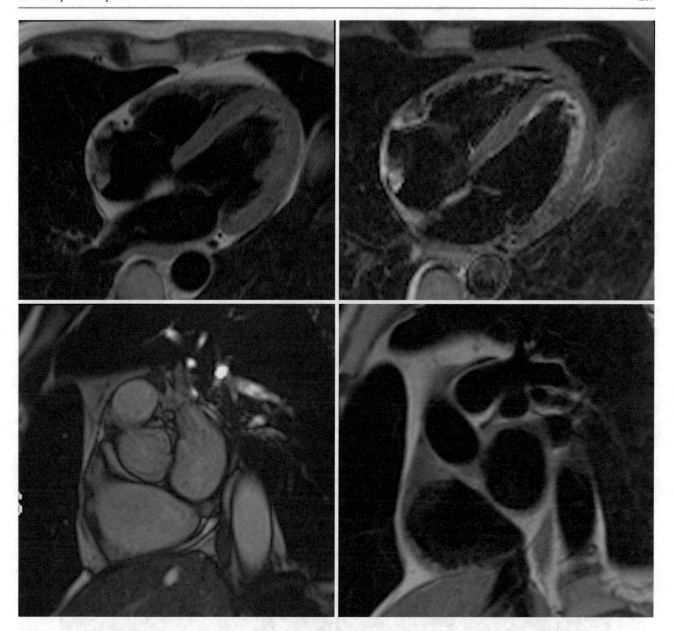

Fig. 8.12 Left upper panel: PDw image in horizontal long axis. Right upper panel: T2w image in horizontal long axis. Left lower panel: SSFP cine images in oblique plane (para-coronal view). Right lower panel, the same plane of the previous image obtained using a PDw sequence

8.7 Loeys-Dietz Syndrome

Medical History Two young relatives with genetic diagnosis of Loeys-Dietz syndrome.

CMR Flowchart Stack of cine images in short-axis view to evaluate biventricular volumes and function. Cine images in oblique view (sagittal and coronal plans) to assess the aortic root and the thoracic Aorta. Cine and phase-contrast images of the aortic valve. Contrast-enhanced 3D angiography (CEMRA) of the thoracic Aorta. LGE images to detect myocardial fibrosis.

Main CMR Findings Normal biventricular volumes and function. No cardiac abnormalities. In both the patients evidence of dilatation of the aortic root.

Patient A: 40 mm (Movie 8.12, Movie 8.13 and Movie 8.14).

Patient B: 47 mm. A: light aortic regurgitation (10%). B: moderate aortic regurgitation (29%) (Movie 8.15, Movie 8.16 and Movie 8.17).

Conclusion In both cases: dilatation of aortic root in Loeys-Dietz syndrome.

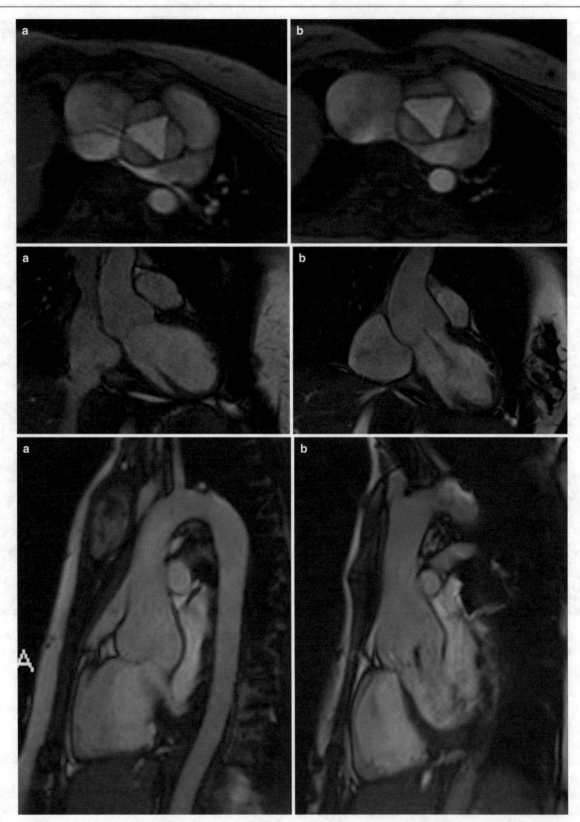

Fig. 8.13 Patient A: left panels; patient B: right panels. Upper panels: cine image in end systole at the level of the aortic valve. Evidence of dilatation of the aortic root in both patients. Middle panels: cine images in coronal plane. Evidence of dilatation of aortic root in both patients. Patient B shows a more significant aortic valve regurgitation. Lower panels: cine images in sagittal plane. Evidence of dilatation of the aortic root in both patients. Patient B shows a more evident aortic valve regurgitation and a more tortuous course of thoracic Aorta resulting in the impossible task to obtain images of the ascending and descending aorta in the same plane

Fig. 8.14 Quantitation of the aortic transvalvular flow. Patient A (upper panel) shows a light aortic valve regurgitation (10%) while patient B (lower panel) shows a moderate regurgitation (29%)

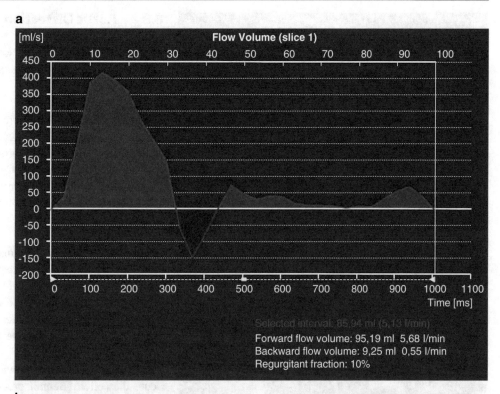

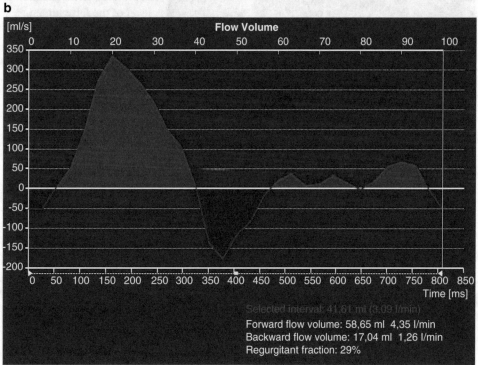

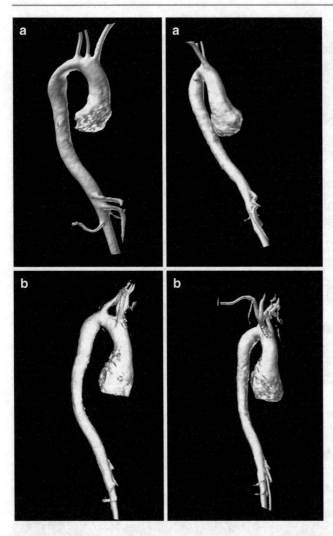

Fig. 8.15 Postcontrast three-dimensional angiography (CEMRA). Both patient A (upper panels) and patient B (lower panels) show dilatation of the aortic root which is more evident in patient B

8.8 Aortic Dissection

Medical History Male, 65 y.o. Previous surgical intervention because of acute type A aortic dissection (Bentall procedure).

CMR Flowchart Stack of cine images in short-axis view to evaluate biventricular volumes and function. Cine images in oblique view (sagittal and coronal plans) to assess the aortic root and the thoracic Aorta. Cine and phase-contrast images of the aortic valve. Contrast-enhanced 3D angiography (CEMRA) of the thoracic Aorta. LGE images to detect myocardial fibrosis/necrosis.

Main CMR Findings Normal biventricular volumes and function. No cardiac abnormalities. Normal morphology of the Bentall prosthesis (Movie 8.18). Evidence of residual dissection at the level of the aortic arch (Movie 8.19 and Movie 8.20). The cross-sectional measurement of flow shows a reduced flow at the level of the false lumen.

Conclusion Successful previous surgical intervention in acute dissection (Bentall procedure). Reduced flow at the level of the false lumen.

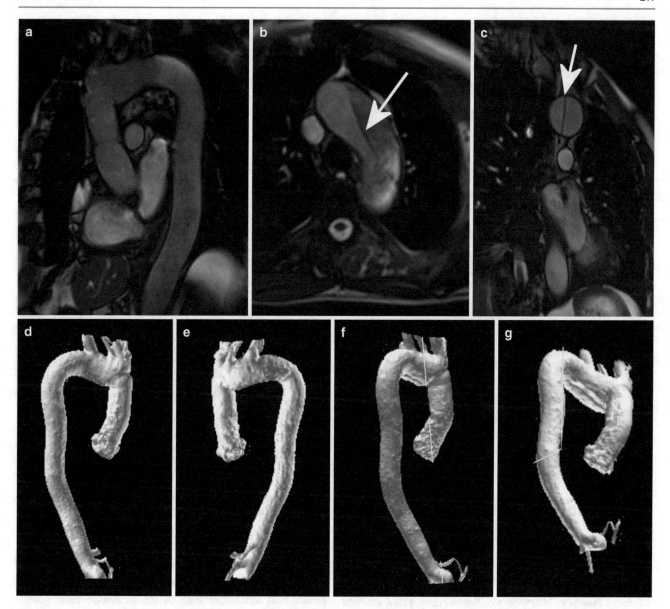

Fig. 8.16 Panel **a**: Still frame from a SSFP cine sequence in oblique view. Normal profile of the vascular conduit in ascending aorta. Panel **b**: still frame from a SSFP cine sequence in axial plane through the aortic arch. The arrow shows the presence of aortic dissection. Panel **c**: still frame from a SSFP cine sequence in cross-sectional view of the aortic arch. The arrow shows the presence of the intimal flap. Panels **d–g**: four views from a three-dimensional contrast angiography showing a morphologic abnormality at the level of the aortic arch

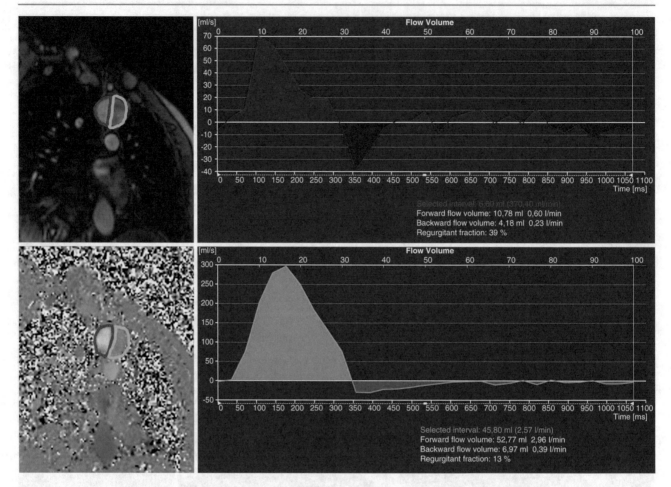

Fig. 8.17 Flow images obtained in cross-sectional view at the level of the aortic arch. Upper left panel: magnitude image. Lower left panel: flow image. Right panels: measurement of flows in the false lumen (upper right panel) and in the true lumen (right lower panel)

8.9   Erdheim-Chester Disease

Medical History Male, 69 y.o. Since many years affected by rheumatic disease. Echocardiographic evidence of chronic pericardial effusion and suspect of para-cardiac tumor. Previous AMI and PTCA stenting.

CMR Flowchart Stack of cine images in short-axis view to evaluate biventricular volumes and function. Cine images in oblique view to assess the localization and dimensions of the para-cardiac mass. T1w, T2w, and LGE images to characterize the para-cardiac mass and assess its eventual infiltrative nature.

Main CMR Findings Normal biventricular volumes and function. Presence of an irregular mass around the right atrium and detectable also in the atrioventricular groove (Movie 8.21 and Movie 8.22). The mass appears to be isointense in T1w and T2w images with respect to the myocardium and shows an active uptake of contrast agent in LGE images. Pericardial effusion. Diffuse involvement of the aortic walls (Movie 8.23).

Conclusion Cardiovascular involvement in Erdheim-Chester disease.

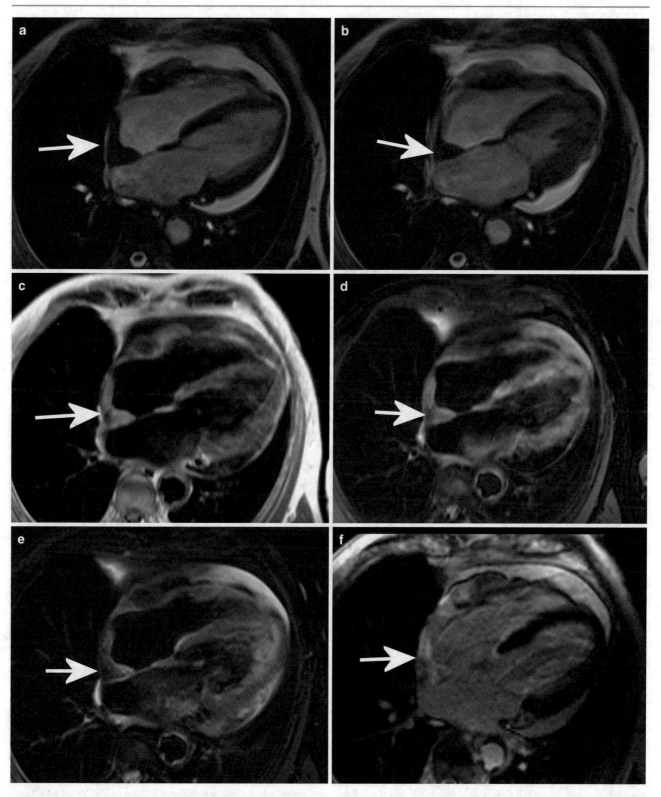

Fig. 8.18 Panels **a** and **b**: still frames in end diastole (**a**) and end systole (**b**) from a SSFP cine sequence in horizontal long axis. The arrows show the para-cardiac mass and the pericardial effusion. Panel **c**: T1w image in horizontal long axis, showing the isointense para-cardiac mass. Panel **d**: T2w fat-saturated image in horizontal long axis, show-ing the isointense para-cardiac mass. Panel **e**: T2w image in horizontal long axis, showing the isointense para-cardiac mass. Panel **f**: LGE image in horizontal long axis showing the active uptake of the contrast agent by the para-cardiac mass

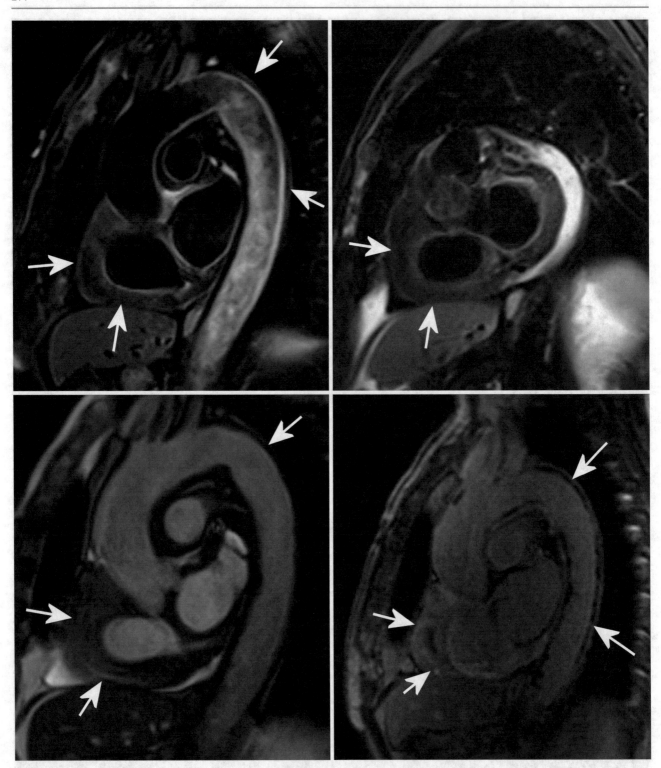

Fig. 8.19 Left upper panel: T1w image in sagittal view. Upper right panel: T2w image in sagittal view. Lower left panel: still frame from SSFP cine sequence in sagittal view. Lower right panel: LGE image in sagittal view. The arrows show the para-cardiac mass at the level of the right atrium and within the atrioventricular grove. Evidence of a diffuse involvement of the aortic walls (arrows)

Bibliography

1. Haller JA Jr, Kramer SS, Lietman SA. Use of CT scans in selection of patients for pectus excavatum surgery: a preliminary report. J Pediatr Surg. 1987;22(10):904–6.

2. Archer JE, Gardner A, Berryman F, Pynsent P. The measurement of the normal thorax using the Haller index methodology at multiple vertebral levels. J Anat. 2016;229(4):577–81.

3. Said SA, Hofman MB, Beek AM, van der Werf T, van Rossum AC. Feasibility of cardiovascular magnetic resonance of angiographically diagnosed congenital solitary coronary artery fistulas in adults. J Cardiovasc Magn Reson. 2007;9(3):575–83.

4. Eroglu AG, Atik SU, Sengenc E, Cig G, Saltik IL, Oztunc F. Evaluation of ventricular septal defect with special reference to the spontaneous closure rate, subaortic ridge, and aortic valve prolapse II. Pediatr Cardiol. 2017;38(5):915–21.

5. Kilner PJ. The role of cardiovascular magnetic resonance in adults with congenital heart disease. Prog Cardiovasc Dis. 2011;54(3):295–304.

6. Lombardi M, Plein S, Petersen S, Bucciarelli-Ducci C, Valsangiacomo-Buechel M, Basso C, Ferrari V. The EACVI textbook of cardiovascular magnetic resonance. Oxford; Oxford University Press; 2018.

7. Mavrogeni S, Bratis K, Karanasios E, Georgakopoulos D, Kaklis S, Varlamis G, Kolovou G, Douskou M, Papadopoulos G. CMR evaluation of cardiac involvement during the convalescence of Kawasaki disease JACC Cardiovasc Imaging 2011;4(10):1140–1.

8. Doan TT, Wilkinson JC, Loar RW, Pednekar AS, Masand PM, Noel CV. Regadenoson stress perfusion cardiac magnetic resonance imaging in children with Kawasaki disease and coronary artery disease. Am J Cardiol. 2019;124(7):1125–32.

9. Bratis K, Chiribiri A, Hussain T, Krasemann T, Henningsson M, Phinikaridou A, Mavrogeni S, Botnar R, Nagel E, Razavi R, Greil G. Abnormal myocardial perfusion in Kawasaki disease convalescence. JACC Cardiovasc Imaging. 2015;8(1):106–8. https://doi.org/10.1016/j.jcmg.2014.05.017.. Epub 2014 Nov 12

10. Altbach MI, Squire SW, Kudithipudi V, Castellano L, Sorrell VL. Cardiac MRI is complementary to echocardiography in the assessment of cardiac masses. Echocardiography. 2007;24(3):286–300.

11. Monwarul Islam AKM, Sayami LA, Zaman S. Chiari network: a case report and brief overview. J Saudi Heart Assoc. 2013;25(3):225–9.

12. Karur GR, Pagano JJ, Bradley T, Lam CZ, Seed M, Yoo SJ, Grosse-Wortmann L. Diffuse myocardial fibrosis in children and adolescents with Marfan syndrome and Loeys-Dietz syndrome. J Am Coll Cardiol. 2018;72(18):2279–81.

13. Loughborough WW, Minhas KS, Rodrigues JCL, Lyen SM, Burt HE, Manghat NE, Brooks MJ, Stuart G, Hamilton MCK. Cardiovascular manifestations and complications of Loeys-Dietz syndrome: CT and MR imaging findings. Radiographics. 2018;38(1):275–86.

14. Sherrah AG, Grieve SM, Jeremy RW, Bannon PG, Vallely MP, Puranik R. MRI in chronic aortic dissection: a systematic review and future directions. Front Cardiovasc Med. 2015;2:5. Published online 2015 Feb 19.

15. Haroche J, Cluzel P, Toledano D, Montalescot G, Touitou D, Grenier PA, Piette JC, Amoura Z. Images in cardiovascular medicine. Cardiac involvement in Erdheim-Chester disease: magnetic resonance and computed tomographic scan imaging in a monocentric series of 37 patients. Circulation. 2009;119(25):e597–8.

Printed in the United States
by Baker & Taylor Publisher Services